May 2006

Best wishes,

Oscar.

Medical Memoirs

Dr J.O.M.C.Craig FRCR, FRCS, FRCP, FRCGP, FRCSI, FFR, RCSI (Hon.) FHKCR (Hon.)

Emeritus Consultant, St Mary's Hospital London W2
Hon. Senior Clinical Lecturer, University of London
Past Director of Clinical Studies, St Mary's Hospital Medical School
Past Director, Department of Radiology, St Mary's Hospital, London W2
Past President Royal College of Radiologists.

Hon. Member Radiological Society of North America.

Medical Memoirs

by

Oscar Craig

The Memoir Club

First published in 2006 by
The Memoir Club
Stanhope Old Hall
Stanhope
Weardale
County Durham

British Library Cataloguing in
Publication Data.
A catalogue record for this book
is available from the
British Library

ISBN: 1-84104-140-8

Typeset by TW Typesetting, Plymouth, Devon
Printed by CPI, Bath

Contents

List of illustrations

Dedication

To Nancy with Love

Coloured crocuses, dancing daffodils
signal spring with soaring spirits,
smiling, sighing, loving.
And she is there.

The warmth of summer in
a beach hut by the sea.
Evening wine in fading light.
And she is there.

Long country walks in golds and browns:
The early autumn chill
that tingles to the bone.
And she is there.

The winter winds with wounding force
bring soundless snow
as treasured Christmas comes to urge us peace.
And she is there.

Spring is no more, no flowers to see.
There is no summer warmth
nor autumn colour or winter's Christmas cheer
without her.

Foreword

Four years ago Oscar Craig published a first volume of autobiography, *A Life in Medicine*, He has now produced a sequel.

Although born in Northern Ireland, he recalls with unalloyed affection his subsequent years in Dublin, where he met his future wife, Nancy, and where he and Nancy qualified in medicine.

A diagnostic radiologist of distinction, he writes of his many activities in the Royal College of Radiologists, of which he became President in 1989; and of his extensive travels, many in the capacity of visiting professor. Of particular interest is the story of the discovery of X-rays and the astounding developments in radiological techniques which have occurred during his professional lifetime. He is unstinting in his praise and affection for his adopted hospital and medical school, St Mary's in Paddington, and he has composed some delightful pen portraits of colleagues there and elsewhere. He also has some pertinent comments to make about the merging of St Mary's with other medical schools, to form but a part of the well named 'empire' of Imperial College.

Despite the fact that he has spent most of his professional life in England, Oscar Craig has never lost his Irishness, and like so many Irishmen he is a great story teller. Furthermore he tells his stories in a highly accessible, anecdotal style, narrative alternating freely with dialogue.

The book starts with a touching, poetic dedication to Nancy. It ends with two especially notable chapters: the first is a reproduction of his Presidential Address to the Harveian Society of London on 'Physicians, Prose and Poetry', about some medical men who became distinguished men of letters; the second is a written version of the Freshers Address which he first delivered to the new intake of students when he became Director of Clinical Studies in 1969, and which he continues to give, by overwhelming popular request, more than twelve years after his retirement.

These are memorable memoirs.

John Ballantyne CBE, FRCS.

Acknowledgements

Ian and Marjory Chapman encouraged me to write, firstly my book, *A Life in Medicine*, and now this sequel. They dispelled my doubts and nourished my hopes. Their interest and professional advice were invaluable.

I'm grateful to many medical colleagues whose friendship I've enjoyed.

I thank Nicolas Coni, editor of the Retired Fellow Society Newsletter of the Royal Society of Medicine, who published articles for me, and gave permission for some to be included in this book, some in Chapter 17, and Harvey celebrations in Chapter 21.

Chapter 1

Northern Ireland

I never met my paternal grandmother. She worked for the firm of Clark and Coates, the cotton barons of Paisley . My father was named James Oscar Max Clark Craig. These were the forenames of Clark. I was named the same. I've never known why. I know nothing of my father's early life. He never spoke of it and I didn't ask. He went to Boston in the United States of America in his twenties with sufficient money to establish a confectionery business. On route to America he stopped in Northern Ireland where he met my mother, Olivia Dowey, in a mutual friend's house where she visited to take tea between teaching classes she gave in Portadown. They met on a few occasions before he sailed. During his seven years away they became engaged. I know nothing of his time in America. He never spoke of it and I didn't ask. During the First World War he decided to come back and booked to sail on the *Lusitania*. He missed the boat. It sailed away as he reached the pier. It was sunk by a submarine with heavy loss of lives. He took another.

My mother said to a friend, 'I won't recognize Jim when he comes off the boat, can you come with me?'

They were on the quayside when the boat came in.

My mother smiled. 'I can see him standing at the rail. I couldn't mistake him.'

Her friend diplomatically slipped away.

On the train to my mother's home in Lurgan, a distance of twenty miles, my father leaned toward her.

'Would you like to read this newspaper?'

He opened another and read for the twenty miles and didn't say a word. She wondered about her future with him and later often told this story. My father was a private man, not given to expressing his opinion lightly and perhaps unable to express his emotions. My mother was talkative, loved company and laughed readily.

When we lived in Belfast life was comfortable. Summer was spent in a house in Bangor by the sea. My mother was skilled at art and painted well in oils.

My father, although untrained, said, 'I could paint as well as you.'

'Don't be ridiculous Jim. How could you, you don't even know how to mix the paints. Don't let anyone hear you brag like that.'

'Well you show me how to mix the paints for the various colours and I'll paint a picture for you.'

She showed him the rudimentary points of colour and mixing. He learnt quickly.

'I want you to take the children to the house in Bangor for some days and when you return I'll have a painting for you.'

It was an excellent oil painting of a ship lying in a bay. My mother was amazed and agreed he had talent. He continued to paint throughout his life apart from one long hiatus in his middle years. Some of his paintings hang in my home. I particularly like his portraits. My mother ceased to paint but those I have seen would match my father's in skill. I never heard him play the violin but he played in an amateur orchestra before I was born. I kept his violin but it was lost on moving house.

When young I spent many holidays in my maternal grandparent's home in Lurgan, where there was a tennis court and stabling for horses. In the house there was the strong religious atmosphere of the Exclusive Brethren. The bible was the dominant book. My grandfather was a small, quiet, gentle, smiling, moustached man held in high regard in the town, and my grandmother grey haired, soft pale skinned, bespectacled, smiling and always dressed in black with a white lace collar. They were old to me. My grandmother ruled her husband, her family and all around from her rocking chair, a study in black not unlike the painting of Whistler's mother. The house was silent and its grave atmosphere was punctuated by the ticking of the grandfather clock in the hall accentuating that time passed slowly.

When my grandmother died, my grandfather in his late seventies came to stay with us for a holiday. I was about nine years old, I remember him saying to me in his bedroom,

'To lose someone you have loved for so long is a terrible tragedy and is so hard to bear.'

I saw the tears roll down his face. Little did I understand then but I feel his pain today. He still stands weeping before me.

One of my aunts married Sandy Foster. My favourite place to stay in Lurgan was in their house. It couldn't have been more different. It was full of fun and controlled disorder. They had two children, Sarita and

Alec. Alec was two years younger than me and Sarita many years older. She and I were fond of each other and later when she went to meet her boyfriends she brought me with her, aged about six. I'm sure they weren't pleased with that, and I think she felt that while I was with her she was safe. We have been close all our lives. She was a very keen golfer and we shared a love of riding.

Aunt Sydney and Uncle Sandy had a caravan in the sand dunes on a long and beautiful beach about twenty miles from Lurgan. One of my earliest memories is rooted there, when I got lost with my cousin. I can still feel the fear of it. I was five but he was only three when I joined them at the caravan. You couldn't see the sea from where it rested among the sand dunes, but you could hear it. That summer was hot and the scent of the thick dune grass was everywhere. I remember the feel of the running silky sand as my feet sank with each step and how I had to pull my foot hard to take another. I loved the sand except when it got into my mouth with a piece of bread. The sand followed me into the caravan and into my bed where it rested on the sheets and joined more sand between my toes. It was friendly then. The dunes were so high that only on the top could you see the next and the hollow between was a haven of silent warmth. There were no other caravans in sight even from the top of the dunes and as far as the eye could see the dunes filled all around and went on and on and on. When I reached the beach it stretched beyond my sight from side to side. I was swallowed by it.

I don't know what made me take his hand and walk away, but the pull of the place and the wish to find more of it over the next dune lured me. Was there something hiding that I couldn't see?

He walked as fast as me but I was older and stronger and took his hand. I helped him climb the dunes and we ran and rolled and laughed down the other side. The sand was in our socks, and in our hair and in our pockets. There was nothing in the hollow but the same silent warmth. I took his hand and we climbed again and again and again. I thought I must have gone in the wrong direction so I turned to the right and held his hand, and then to the left and held his hand. Still nothing new appeared and one dune and hollow was like the other. It was fun but how tired I was getting. He said nothing. I knew I must go back, but we rested for a while. He said nothing. I took his hand to the top of the dune to see the caravan. I saw the stretch of dunes, farther than ever before, higher than ever before, more alike than ever before, but I could see no caravan. I didn't know which way to walk but I knew I would see the caravan from the next dune. I took his hand but I saw nothing but sand and grass. I tried the next, and the next and the next.

It takes but a moment for happiness to change and fear crept over my body numbing my senses. I was lost forever. He said nothing. I couldn't stop the tears as he smiled at me, but I didn't tell him we were lost. I cried for quite a time, sitting on the sand and holding his hand. He said nothing.

The man said, 'Hello, why are you crying? You're a big boy.'

I told him I was five. He said, 'Your brother isn't crying.'

I said, 'He's my cousin.'

He brought us to the caravan.

It's surprising that my Aunt Sydney with her Exclusive Brethren background married Uncle Sandy, as his American father owned the cinema in Lurgan. None of my grandparents' children dared go to a cinema. It was considered by the Brethren to be a place inhabited by the devil and his disciples. Despite this the youngest of my uncles, who still lived at home, crept into the projection box of the cinema where he couldn't be seen. He watched the film through the window sitting on a high stool. I was there often as I loved the place. The projector made a rhythmic whirling sound and the light from it danced in the room before shooting to the screen through the air filled with the unusual sweet smell of film. I can hear the sound and taste the smell as I write and the image of the projection room is vivid, comfortable and warm. The film had to be rewound and cleaned by hand on a roller and I often did this. I learnt to thread the films into the projector and during the film to change from one projector to another. I was only about nine or ten years old. I'm sure everything is automatic today but I wonder if it is as much fun. My Uncle Sandy was in charge of the cinema and he and I were firm friends even at that tender age. This mutual respect continued throughout our lives.

I have loved films all my life. I had screen role models. I'm sure they shaped my behaviour and even my ambitions. Such is the power of the screen. Lew Ayers when he played Dr Kildare strengthened my resolve to study medicine. Walter Pidgeon displayed a personality I wished to mimic. I wanted to marry a girl like Greer Garson, especially in her role as Mrs Miniver. When she and Walter Pidgeon played together in

Madame Curie, I was in seventh heaven. My first date with Nancy, who was to become my wife, was to the films. We saw *Madame Curie*. Even in my mature years I was influenced. When I saw Spencer Tracy in *Guess Who's coming to Dinner*, I wanted to grow old in his fashion. I know about his off screen life and his drinking which I don't want to copy.

There was less violence in the films before the Second World War and sex was assumed but not seen. Remember the tide coming in and out! At an early age my feelings about the opposite sex were clothed in awe and mystery. Perhaps they still are.

The comfort of going to my uncle's cinema was to change into one of excitement and adventure when war began in 1939. By that time my family had moved to Dublin, but I still spent holidays in Lurgan. Northern Ireland was full of troops of both the United Kingdom and the United States of America. I was twelve when the war began. In Northern Ireland I loved seeing the uniforms of the men and women of the forces, the army lorries, tanks, jeeps, bombers, fighter planes, anti-aircraft guns, barrage balloons and all the paraphenalia of war. Northern Ireland also had the 'black out' which added to the excitement. Uniformed men and women packed my uncle's cinema nightly. It all seemed so romantic. The films portrayed romance, valour and 'on our side' exemplary behaviour. I didn't see the dark side of war or human behaviour. The truth of war would have been crippling for everyone.

Aunt Sydney opened her home to soldiers whom she entertained with her outgoing kindness. My cousin Sarita married a young soldier, Ray Taylor, just before he embarked for Italy. Both Ray and Sarita were to play an important part in my life in London. When Nancy and I qualified in medicine we stayed in their house in London while looking for our first professional posts. Much was to happen before that however. One of Ray's soldier buddies, Alan Bolton from London, was friendly with my sister Maxime. Maxime and Alan were witnesses when Nancy and I married in 1950. Ray and Sarita were sailing in the Mediterranean in their cruiser.

Life in Lurgan changed enormously during the war. This little town, with its many churches, its strong non-conformist attitudes, its insular philosophy and its ridiculous divide between Protestant and Catholic was turned upside down. It seemed it would never be quite the same again, but it's sad that religious prejudice did survive, as we have witnessed in the past decades. Such is the intransigence of the Orange heritage and Catholicism. I despair about this.

My Uncle Charlie owned a large farm on which he kept herds of cattle. He was a successful man and had a butcher's shop to sell his beef, thus omitting a middle man.

His son, John, was sensitive, ambitious and competitive. He began working with his father but they were so different it couldn't last. Uncle Charlie was blunt, self assured and dictatorial. He was also paranoid, especially regarding the Ministry of Agriculture, and indeed any government in power. Often I heard him say, 'The government is after me again. These new regulations are planned just to destroy me. They are after my money, and when they get it they waste it.' He believed this passionately.

Any bond that existed between John and his father was shattered when John bought a farm of his own, stocked it with a prize herd and sold his meat in opposition to his father. However both survived. John liked the good life. He was fond of clothes and dressed immaculately in tailored suits and hand-made shoes. My father wore hand-made shoes in his wealthy period. My life in medicine has been successful but I've never been able to afford hand-made shoes. Perhaps the truth is I've spent money in other ways. When we lived in Dublin John Dowey often visited us. He bought cattle in Southern Ireland and transported them to Northern Ireland. I remember him in evening dress going to dinners and dances in Dublin. He gave me my first 'tails'. When I was a medical student money was in short supply and the gift of John's cast-off 'tails' was very welcome. There was one problem. John had a congenital dislocation of the hip and his left leg was shorter than the right. I adjusted the trousers by having my braces long on the right and shorter on the left. I'm convinced nobody noticed any discrepancy.

It was on my Uncle Charlie's farm that I began riding. I learnt to saddle a horse but had no formal lessons. I just mounted and rode. As a result my riding is unschooled, but I've continued riding all my life. My sister Maxime was a poor rider. I have a sharp image of her returning one evening when the horse bolted to its stable and she ducked just in time to prevent her head being removed by the top of the stable door. I too had my problems. My Uncle Dick was a keen huntsman and an excellent horseman. In fact I think he was the best horseman I've met. When I went with him on my first hunt I had a pair of releasing stirrups. I jumped a ditch and the ground on the other side was wet and soft. It fell away on landing and my horse stumbled. I fell off but one of the stirrups failed to release and I was lying helplessly on my back with my left foot in the stirrup high on the horse. We were in a wood. I knew the horse to be excitable as I'd ridden him often and he would shy if a piece of paper fluttered on the ground. Fortunately my uncle was riding just ahead, saw the fall and came back. He approached gently and grabbed the reins, dismounted and released me.

My father owned bakeries and confectionery shops in Belfast. In 1934, I was seven when he lost his business. I never knew why, but I was told it was the result of the great financial depression of the time. This may have been so, but as I grew older I realized my father was not suited to a life in business. He was unable to make hard decisions based on financial gain; he was a kind man with an artistic temperament.

He took a job as manager of a bakery in Dublin which didn't suit him either, but the financial success was in the end not solely his responsibility. He had to work very hard and the change in lifestyle was enormous for him and the whole family. It must have been very difficult for them but as I was only seven, it meant little to me. I had two sisters, Jean aged twelve and Maxime aged seventeen at the time.

Maxime was the one most upset and the fall from financial and social security never left her. Her resentment remained into adult life and explained many of her characteristics. She was cursed and blessed by an extraordinary feeling of importance, resting in herself and her immediate family. Often when telling us of a disagreement with a saleswoman, she would say, 'I don't think she knew who I was.' This sad attitude made us laugh. She was a difficult woman all her life but had sterling qualities, dependable, loyal, outrageously honest in her opinions even to the point of hurtful, intelligent and capable of great love. She was engaged to a law student throughout his student days, who after seven years jilted her. She never married. During the Second World War she enlisted in the Navy, Army and Air Force Institution (NAAFI). She was a manageress and very successful in the post. Not being born to earn her living in the market place, in her eyes, she took up nursing and when over thirty studied to became a midwife in London. She became a sister in a local hospital in Surrey. She was in the mould of the old fashioned ward sisters and regretfully was often feared by the patients. However she did well. She lived with my wife and me for many years in London. Maxime developed a reticulosis from which she died in her sixties. She loved our children and we still miss her.

My sister Jean couldn't have been more different. Jean was popular with the boys in both Dublin and Belfast. She loved the social life, tennis, dancing and parties. At an early age she had a gift for interior design and was employed for a time in designing window displays for prestigious shops. After numerous boyfriends she choose Norman Page, a hunting, shooting and fishing man in Donacloney, Northern Ireland, the son of the local 'squire'. He became a textile engineer. They married and moved to Leeds in Yorkshire. They both missed the life of Irish country gentry, and their love of Ireland, which remained their spiritual home, never left them. I understand that. Jean's ability at interior design never faltered and she converted many houses with admirable taste.

Unfortunately my sisters, not surprisingly, were not soulmates and as a child I was distressed to hear them clash so often. Regretfully this continued into adult life and when both were together the atmosphere was tense.

My mother was a kind, soft hearted, loving woman who was constantly anxious. She had been a teacher of domestic science in her young days. Perhaps her anxiety was initiated by our loss of wealth, but I think it was inborn as I too inherited it.

My father was the classic dour Scot. He spoke little and to my regret we never had a meaningful conversation together all my life. If only I could talk to him now. How many sons must have said this of their fathers? He had a temper and I think there were times when I was afraid of him. I know he was full of concern for me and I remember well when short of money we needed new shoes and he paid more for mine than for his. I also remember when I was a medical student I attended a party with a beautiful girl and arrived home as he was leaving for work. I met him in the drive and was anxious about my reception. He smiled and said, 'Good morning', and walked on. I owe them both so much as they encouraged me when I wished to study medicine, for which everything had to be paid in those days. When, approaching retirement, they had little money and the prospect of a very small pension, Nancy and I were established in London. We invited them to come to London and live with us. They did for eighteen years. I had discussed this with Nancy before our marriage. It turned out that Nancy was the rock on which our subsequent house and home were built.

Chapter 2

Dublin

My father's loss in business in Belfast and our move to Dublin would be considered by many as a disaster. It was the best thing that could have happened to me, and I long to believe that God works in wondrous ways, so often only understandable in retrospect.

I think the relative absence of money taught me to spend it carefully and later in life to appreciate having some. A fault it may have encouraged is that I had little interest in making it, confident I would survive without it. This was a form of arrogance. Nancy in later years would find outdated cheques in my jacket. I've changed in retirement! Perhaps the most important benefit I had from the move to Dublin was to have my formative years in Southern Ireland. Here I found a totally different culture to that in Northern Ireland.

Belfast is an industrial city. Its wealth lay in its shipbuilding, its engineering, factories of all kinds and a strong linen industry. During the war the factories multiplied to supply arms to the British Armed Forces and its wealth increased.

The inhabitants of Northern Ireland were basically Scottish, sent to occupy the land for political reasons. They brought with them a laudable work ethos, but also a piety that fuelled a narrow religious zeal. This curse continues and grows as we have witnessed in these past decades.

Although Belfast is not a beautiful city, it is surrounded by picturesque countryside. The Ards peninsula which I visited recently is hard to beat for beauty. Green lush fields cascade to an exciting coastline with rocky coves and inviting beaches. Sailing is a way of life along this coast and the yachts dance in the waves, their masts' rigging singing to allure the native and visitor to the sport. However even with this relief I find the stern Presbyterian ethos suffocating. It was here in a Northern village that a relative by marriage hid the Sunday newspaper under his coat, not to be thought reading other than the bible on this holy day. I'm glad not to have grown in such a repressed society. But the farms are clean and prosperous and there was little financial suffering in the cities.

South of the border, there were pubs and poverty, but prose and poetry were more important than the pound. Southern Ireland had no Presbyterian ethos, but Protestants, including Presbyterians, were welcomed and cared for. One of the first Presidents of the Republic of Ireland was Douglas Hyde, a Protestant, and another was Erskine Childers. I went to school with the son of the Jewish Lord Mayor of Dublin. I didn't witness, feel or suffer from any religious prejudice growing up in Dublin, in this Catholic country. I loved being there within the carefree, live for today, enjoy the minute, laugh or drown your troubles, atmosphere.

The city of Dublin stretches around Dublin Bay with the shape of a horseshoe. The quayside is close to the city centre. The River Liffey passes through O'Connell Street, Dublin's wide central thoroughfare. It's a tidal river and not attractive in the city when the tide is out. Nelson, a figure of British power and colonial rule, towered over Dublin on a pillar as high as that in Trafalgar Square. It was placed centrally in O'Connell Street, with the statues of Parnell at one end and O'Connell at the other, both champions of Ireland's struggle for independence. Nelson's presence in this position didn't seem bizarre to me, as aged seven I knew nothing of the rebellion. Some years after I left Dublin a bomb removed Nelson. Although I have great regard for Nelson and have a print of him in my dining room and another in my study in Cheam, I cannot weep for his removal from such a prominent place in Dublin's main street. Queen Victoria's statue at one time sat in front of the Dail, Ireland's parliament building. Quietly this was removed to another site.

There are some new statues. A modern statue of a mythical Anna Livia sits in a fountain in O'Connell Street. It was referred to, by the Dubliners, as 'the floosie in the Jacuzzi'. After repeated interference the fountain was removed. There are statues of James Joyce and Molly Malone. Older classical statues of the past remain and two of my favourites stand outside Trinity College: Burke, the Irish born English statesman and champion of Irish Catholics on the left, and Goldsmith the Irish born poet, playwright and novelist on the right.

Dublin is a beautiful Georgian city. However on the outskirts of the city many squares with their British architecture tumbled into slums. The inhabitants were a pitiful sight with large families crowded into single rooms. Prams and bottles fought for space and black shawled women gossiped in the broken doorways while their menfolk lounged in the streets finding no work in this new republic devoid of an industrial heritage. This was part of the price for independence. Fortunately the poverty of the south has gone, but I remember the distressing conditions in the slums when I did my obstetrics and delivered babies in their homes.

There is beauty in College Green where Trinity College faces the majesty of the Bank of Ireland, which in 1728 was the new Parliament building. Another fine building is the Royal College of Surgeons, in St Stephen's Green where I studied medicine.

During the rebellion Countess Markievich and her troops in home-made green uniforms made a stand in the College, and the bullet marks of the battle remain around its imposing front.

When I lived in Dublin, students and bicycles were everywhere. Today there are more cars, but students still flock to Dublin and pack the coffee houses interspersed between stylish shops in Grafton Street. Street musicians are plentiful but often unorthodox. I remember one elderly gentleman and his wife, both of genteel birth, playing the harp and violin in Grafton Street. They became part of the Dublin scene at the time and part of the backcloth of the city. This is a city of conversation. In Dublin there is no lack of it. Much talk is made sitting over coffee or porter. Is it surprising that four Nobel Prize winners lived here, Shaw, Yeats, Beckett and in 1995 Seamus Heaney? Three literary giants, Oscar Wilde, Sean O'Casey and James Joyce, surely deserved similar acclaim.

It has taken years for Southern Ireland to shake off the yoke of its political past but as part of the European Union it is now more outward looking and bursting with energy and confidence. An extract from a newsletter written by the Medical Society of London recently reports, 'Dublin has overtaken Amsterdam and Prague as the most popular weekend destination in Europe. A city of great cultural and historical interest, the booming economy, the emergence of a confident contemporary architecture and the asset of having the youngest population in Europe, have made Dublin one of the most transformed cities in the world'. It's over fifty years since I lived there before this transformation but my memories of Dublin are happy. I hope the new-found commercial wealth won't effect the wealth it has in music, literature, theatre and the arts.

My prep school in Dublin was the school of the Clontarf Presbyterian Church. Mr McIvor the headmaster, a worthy member of the church, was a formidable man. He was a typical practising Presbyterian, honest, hard-working, reliable, conservative, orthodox and a strict disciplinarian. My memory is dominated by the right-hand back pocket of his trousers, where he kept a short thick wooden stick, used to inflict punishment on the hands of the pupils that displeased him. The fear began if you saw his right hand go like a flash behind his back. It reappeared just as quickly with the dreaded weapon which he flicked from his wrist with remarkable skill, honed from years of experience. It was rarely just one strike. Three was the average. I was a talkative boy, a defect in young and mature years. On one occasion Mr McIvor said, 'The next boy that talks in class will receive just punishment.' The boy next to me said, 'Ah sure he's good at that.'

Mr McIvor looked in our direction and fast as a leopard was standing in front of me raising the proverbial woodpiece. I longed to cry out, 'It wasn't me,' but I said nothing before or after the unjust punishment. I look back with pride on keeping my mouth shut. There were many times as an adult when I should have remembered this valuable lesson.

The form master was equally terrifying. He merely threatened without inflicting harm, but you always lived under the threat and could never be sure. He carried the classical bamboo cane and on entering the class placed it in full view on his desk, while removing his jacket and rolling up his sleeves. This had a profound effect on young boys. I don't think it did any harm. Certainly nobody needed counselling.

Teachers were in control and not criticized by parents, or the public at large, and never by the press, for imposing harsh discipline.

The minister of that church is the first minister I remember. He was the Reverend Doctor Morrow. I can still see him walk from the vestry, at the back of the church, up the aisle to the imposing pulpit, correctly placed above the congregation and to one side of the organ and choir. He was an imposing figure, dressed in his gown with its coloured hood, high clerical collar and starched clerical bands. His silver hair was long, brushed back to flow down his neck, wavy and shining to reflect light.

Above his white bushy moustache was a long straight nose. His gait was purposeful, looking neither to right or left he walked confidently to his rightful place in the pulpit.

Here was a man of substance whose kind eyes disguised the stern will that dominated the church and the community. This was a leader, surely the role of all men of the cloth. There are few of his calibre today. More's the pity. When he found out that one of my hobbies was collecting clay pipes he gave me a Meershaum pipe he had smoked for years. I prized it.

The church was always full. The congregation sat silently and immobile in shining wooden pews, breathing quietly the polish-laden air. Men and women wore dark clothes, the men three-piece suited, from the most affluent to the church caretaker. Every woman wore a hat. It would have been a mortal sin for a woman not to wear a hat and none would have dared enter without one. I remember a young couple appear one Sunday and to my surprise the man was wearing a large double breasted light fawn overcoat of remarkably good quality. His wife was dressed fashionably in a bright two piece suit, high heeled shoes and wore a jaunty feathered hat which hugged her head of smooth blonde hair. Her makeup was dominated by bright ruby lips. I loved them immediately. They were the first break with tradition I had seen there. I thought they looked so attractive and maybe I could grow up like him and marry a girl like her. They were such a contrast to the congregation I was sure they would never come back. I was wrong. I never knew who they were or from where they came but they had money, status and influence and were accepted readily by the upper middle class elders and congregation. I saw them each week.

I was a trouble-maker in Sunday school, and led the gang. Many Sunday school teachers had a hard time with me and my boisterous antics. An easy disruption was to keep changing places in class and I persuaded the other boys to do the same. This caused pandemonium. I remember driving one kind elderly man to distraction. I think my behaviour was conditioned by the strict discipline of everyday school at the time, but I'm ashamed of my behaviour now.

Following Sunday school we went into church and it must have irritated the Sunday teachers to see me sing in the choir, often solo, fair haired, scrubbed and innocent, deceiving many in the congregation. The organist and choir master was Matthew (Matty) Taylor, who thought I had a good voice worth encouraging. He trained me enthusiastically and spent a great deal of time with me. A civil servant by profession he was a thin delicate nervous man with a wispy moustache, prominent teeth and wore round horn-rimmed spectacles. He dressed well, with no flair, but played the organ magnificently. He had a beautiful young wife. They had no children and I wonder if I was a substitute. I spent a great deal of time with them.

I remember when aged nine I cried for some reason or another she cuddled me. I enjoyed it.

Matty Taylor did much for my singing, encouraging me and giving me solo performances. It must have been hurtful to him when a neighbouring church enticed me to sing in their choir. My parents shouldn't have permitted this. On offer were even more solo parts with more extensive publicity and I was encouraged to take this opportunity. It led to harsh words between Matty Taylor and my father. I regret all this, but I was too young to influence matters. It was wrong and should never have happened. However shortly after this I obtained a scholarship into St Andrew's College and this in itself would have caused a change. My voice broke within two years.

St Andrew's College was a boarding and day school for upper middle class Protestant boys. It was highly thought of in Dublin and had a good academic reputation. I was good at languages, Latin, French and Gaelic, but poor in mathematics, physics and geography. I would like to have had a better schooling in literature, prose and poetry, but this was perhaps my fault. I wish I had a better knowledge of European history. I was very happy at St Andrew's and played rugby, joined the boxing club and the Boy Scouts Troop. I made many friends and was one of the 'in crowd'.

My progress in class was sufficient to get me into medical school. Since the age of seven I knew I would study medicine. I cannot say why.

I had few teachers that impressed me and I regret none was a role model. They were all however kind and conscientious. The headmaster, Mr Southgate, was a pleasant Englishman, who was accompanied everywhere by his dalmation dog, called Peter. Little did he know how often we planned attacks on that dog but never carried them out. One of our best teachers was Mr Lyons, who taught French but disappointed us by leaving to take a lecturer's post at Oxford University. The teacher we knew best was Mr Ferguson, our sports master. Fergie was young, keen and an archetypal teacher. In any century, in any circumstances, in any country he would be a teacher. He was also our Scoutmaster. We were an unruly troop of scouts. On one occasion when camping in a large estate in Drogheda, Fergie caught us having a 'rough house' late at night in a tent. He knew the likely ring leaders immediately and pointed to us.

'You, you and you won't be having breakfast in the morning.'

'Ah sir, that isn't fair.'

'I'm not talking about what's fair. I'm saying you won't be having breakfast. Is that understood?'

'Yes sir.'

In the morning, Mr Thorpe, a student from Oxford University on a teaching elective, met us in the field outside the tent. He had heard about the incident.

'Are you hungry?'

'Starving, sir.'

'I'm going into the village. Come with me.'

'Yes sir.'

In the village he stopped at a sweet shop. 'Stay outside,'

He returned in a few minutes. 'There are bars of chocolate on the counter. I'm not giving them to you, but if you go inside you can pick them up.'

He left us and walked back to the camp. We followed later, but not so hungry. We wished he wouldn't go back to Oxford after the holiday, but he did. We never met again.

Mr Buchanan was the master we respected and feared most; a man of few words and great authority. We were surprised and pleased when he married the matron. We thought them old, but they were middle-aged, perhaps in their late forties. I played rugby badly and cricket even worse but was good at boxing. When I was in hospital practice this topic came up at a dinner party in my home. When the subject of professional boxing came up I spoke of my boxing at school. This led to a remark from a colleague, a psychiatrist.

'I'm not surprised Oscar, you're aggressive.'

'Who, me?'

'Yes.'

'You can't be serious.'

'Of course I am.'

I was so upset I nearly hit him!

I remember my first big fight aged twelve. I had been coached and trained well by Billy. He was a small man, thin and wiry, with a square face and close cropped hair. As he walked he seemed to glide through the air so light was he on his feet. He only spoke to bark commands, but he was regarded by all as friendly. Billy had been a champion in the British Army. The large tattoo on his chest was the Union flag and on his back the British coat of arms. These were the reasons why in those days he never removed his vest in the Republic of Ireland. He no longer fought in tournaments because of his age but loved his job as the College boxing coach. The masters in their gowns and mortar boards were respected and feared, but Billy in his vest and shorts was admired. He loved his daughter Moira more than the noble art of boxing, but nothing else. Moira played the accordion and Billy couldn't understand that the sports master declined his offer for her to play at school functions. The boys would have loved it. I remember Billy with great affection and he remains one of the characters in my life whose image appears clearly in my mind sixty three years later. I was aware I was one of his favourites and he gave me special attention. During training the bigger boys frequently hurt me in bouts but Billy was careful to see that I wasn't significantly injured.

As the day approached for our match against St Jude's School, the training intensified and my excitement grew as I anticipated my first appearance in a boxing contest in public. It was going to be especially significant as my father was going to be in a ringside seat.

For a boxer I was slight in build, thin and without any visible muscle. I could never win by brute force so had to develop other skills. I could think and move quickly and could see an opening in my opponent's guard in a flash. Billy had taught me well. He had taught me to use what strength I had by putting all my body weight behind each blow, moving forward into my opponent. Using my weight in this fashion produced a blow of surprising force considering my sparse build. My greatest asset however was my speed and during the months leading up to the fight I trained hard to improve my stamina. However I had noticed that each blow I received sapped me of energy and my search for breath and strength became critical. I was not built to take many strong punches.

My father came with me to the gymnasium on the night. He was silent and said nothing to me when he left to go to his seat, but I knew he wished me well and was enjoying the atmosphere and the excitement. In the communal changing room I watched the boys from

St Jude's arrive and each of us searched for his opponent. Mine looked bigger and stronger than me. In my future bouts this always seemed to be the case. It was at this first view of my opponent that the fear began. I searched his face for any sign of weakness or any hint that he too might be afraid. I found none, and he was smiling; my fear intensified. I'm talkative by nature but as I changed I was silent. Billy bound my hands with the tapes, the first of many times to come. He noticed my silence.

'Are you alright?'

I couldn't tell him I was frightened. He left me to go to the ring for the earlier bouts. As the time grew near for my bout the fear also grew but I began to feel an excitement I'd never known before. I've wondered many times how I could feel fear and yet at the same time be exhilarated. I walked to the ring and it seemed I wasn't there but watching myself do it. I was aware of the regular rhythmic thumping of my heart against my chest, faster and stronger than usual. I wondered if people could hear it. Why was my mouth so dry? Although I could see the packed gymnasium I couldn't see individual faces. The room was dominated by the brightness in the ring. If ever there was no turning back this was it. I went toward the corner where Billy was standing and he held the ropes apart for me to enter. His face was friendly and smiling. I could hardly believe I was doing this. I could see my opponent in his corner, still smiling. I couldn't smile. Billy had my favourite black gloves which he held for me as I slipped my hand into each, first the right and then the left. This ritual intensified the overpowering thrill of the moment, the seriousness of the task ahead and the determination to win with glory. Years later I was to get a similar thrill when putting my hands into surgical gloves, but for more noble reasons and without the fear.

The names of the fighters and the weights were announced. Billy tapped my head.

'Do your best. You'll be alright.'

The bell rang. Everything changed. My fear had gone. There was only one person before me and I saw none other. My task was clear. I moved quickly into the centre of the ring remembering Billy's words never to be caught on the ropes. I stared into my opponent's eyes and as I had learnt would never take my eyes off his. It was from his eyes I would read his intentions. In these first few moments it was necessary to analyse him, find his weakness, judge his strength and at the same time establish my authority. As Billy had taught me I moved forward hitting with a straight left to his face. These punches hit the mark time after time. I was doing well. His defence was to tie me up in a clinch. He lay on my body and his weight took away some of my strength. He started to come in close to me, where I was unable to hit him with my straight left punches, and he caught me with powerful blows to my head and body. He kept coming into me and clinching when I tried to move away. My God, I realized he was much stronger than me. Suddenly I was caught by a sledgehammer blow to the side of my face. The energy flew from my body and the power from my legs. It was my turn to hang on to him for dear life, tying up his arms. My mind was in a turmoil and I thought I would fall to the floor.

The referee separated us but he was immediately back in close, catching me with rapid blows. I was in extreme danger. In those seconds of mental and physical pain I saw the fight being lost. Fortunately the bell sounded for the end of the first round. I moved toward my corner knowing how dangerous this opponent was, and realizing the truth I'd been told, that the boxing ring is the loneliest place in the world.

As I sat on my stool, Billy barked in my ear, 'No close quarters, keep moving, use your speed, in and out quickly, straight lefts, move, move.'

In the second round I moved faster throwing straight lefts and fast right jabs, then moved quickly before he could clinch. I kept moving and he couldn't get close enough to tie me up. At no time did he find me standing in the same place. I circled him, struck him and moved to his side. His counter-blows struck air as I had moved again, to the left, the right or straight back. He never knew which way I'd move. His face no longer smiled and his eyes which I held fixed to mine lacked lustre. He was getting weaker, and any blows that reached me carried none of their former strength. I was now enjoying this and was upset when the bell sounded for the end of the round as I wanted to finish him off.

As I sat in the corner, Billy was pleased.

'You've got him. Keep on the same. Straight lefts, fast in and out, keep moving.'

When the bell went for the third round I was fast off my stool and bounding across the ring toward him. He had lost any ability to stop my blows to his head and body, and soon failed to counter them. I forced him back to the ropes where I hit him to the head quite at will, his defence gone. Suddenly his hands fell to his side. I was startled. What's he doing. He's open wide. I prepared to give him the final crushing blow, but looking into his eyes, I saw despair, defeat and anguish. I couldn't do it. I stood back as the referee jumped between us. I was awarded a technical knockout.

Billy undid my gloves in the corner as the verdict was announced. He was smiling broadly, as he ruffled my hair shouting, 'Well done, well done.'

I changed and joined my father. He said nothing about the fight then or later.

However his eyes were bright and shiny.

I've wondered all my life why I didn't deliver that final crushing blow.

Years later and after many boxing bouts I went to medical school and my boxing ceased. The reason was my preoccupation with study and other pursuits such as music. I sang as a bass baritone in choirs and in solo parts in concerts. I'm glad I stopped boxing. It's a very exciting sport but dangerous, and now I think, ugly. I've learnt the dangers of repeated damage to the brain from blows to the head. Each blow causes the brain to hit against the dense skull wall and small (petechial) haemorrhages occur. These can be seen with Computed Tomography (CT) scanning and Magnetic Resonance Imaging. These haemorrhages can affect long term mental ability. If a large haemorrhage occurs it's life threatening. This is liable to happen if there is congenital blood vessel weakness. These defects can remain unknown until some catastrophe occurs. Despite the fun I had from boxing I would not recommend it as either an amateur or professional sport. However my boxing medals were made into a bracelet for Nancy. We loved that bracelet and were upset when it was stolen from our home.

CHAPTER 3

The Discovery of X-Rays

MOST OF MY MEDICAL CAREER has been spent in the specialty of clinical radiology, following some earlier medical posts. I qualified at the Royal College of Surgeons in Ireland in 1950, as did Nancy Burleigh, my girl friend. We sailed to Liverpool and took the train to London. We both took posts in general practice in separate but close practices, and married on 12th August 1950. The following year I took a house surgeon's post in St Helier Hospital, Carshalton. Returning to general practice for a further two years I was then called to do my National Service. I did this in the Royal Air Force and was posted to the RAF Hospital in Ely, Cambridgeshire, where I studied for my Fellowship in Surgery. I obtained this and left the Air Force, though still uncertain what medical future to follow. I obtained an appointment as Resident House Surgeon to Professor Ian Aird at the Hammersmith Hospital, London. It was here that I decided on my future career. I was impressed by the work of Professor Robert Steiner and Dr John Laws, both clinical radiologists. Their skills and expertise in diagnosis was central to the treatment of patients and indeed to the management of clinical disorders involving all specialties. I was especially fired by the developments in cardiac and vascular investigations which although still in their infancy in the early 1950s were making surgical treatments safer and more effective. I spoke to Robert Steiner who advised me to apply for trainee posts in clinical radiology. I was fortunate in obtaining one at St Mary's Hospital, Paddington. Nancy continued in general practice and supported me while I specialized. At this stage I had been qualified seven years. Having obtained my Fellowship in Radiology, in 1963, I was appointed Consultant in Clinical Radiology to the Department of Radiology, at St Mary's. I had then been qualified thirteen years.

It is interesting to record the early development of clinical radiology. This story is familiar to many but my account is based on the book, *Pioneers and Early Years, a History of British Radiology* by E.H. Burrows published in 1986. Much of this text belongs to Burrows.

X-rays were discovered by William Conrad Roentgen. He was the son of a Dutch mother and a German father, who were cousins. He was born in Dusseldorf in the Rhineland in 1845, but when he was three the family moved to Utrecht in the Netherlands where Roentgen lived for the next seventeen years. He had the reputation of being a trouble-maker and when one of his classmates drew a caricature of a teacher he got the blame, his classmate remaining silent. Roentgen was expelled. This seems a harsh treatment even for those times and I wonder what else might have been against him. His school reports were good, but strangely the only bad marks he ever got were in physics. The remarks written on his physics report were 'Zeer slecht', which translates as 'very bad'. Roentgen never matriculated and couldn't be admitted to a university. He went to a Polytechnic in Zurich and when 23 years old got a diploma in mechanical engineering. He became a protégé of August Kundt, a physicist, and abandoned his mechanical engineering for physics. In June 1869 he obtained a PhD in physics. In 1870 Kundt moved to Wurzburg as Professor and applied for university status for Roentgen. This was rejected as the university said he hadn't had a satisfactory schooling in Latin and Greek. Roentgen nonetheless worked as Kund's assistant for eighteen years, and eventually was appointed Professor of Physics in Wurzburg in 1888.

Philipp Lenard, a physicist born in Bratislava, trained in Budapest and Vienna, worked in Germany and was investigating cathode rays in 1893. He identified rays which at the time were called Lenard rays, and indeed he was very close to the discovery of X-rays. Lenard published the results of his work in October 1895. Roentgen borrowed a vacuum tube from Lenard but in fact having decided to pursue Lenard's work used a different tube, a Hittorf-Crookes tube, for his experiments.

Late in the afternoon of Friday 8th November 1895, Roentgen wrapped the vacuum tube in black cardboard, turned off the lights and turned on an electric current through the tube. A cardboard screen coated in barium platinocyanide was lying some feet away. He noticed a fluorescence on the screen, a soft glow which puzzled him.

He cut off the current and the glow disappeared. He started the current and the glow reappeared. He was aware he was looking at something entirely new and unknown to any living scientist. (My thoughts jump to another chance finding many years later when Alexander Fleming observed the effects of mould on the bacteria growing on an agar plate in his laboratory at St Mary's Hospital, London.) Roentgen remained late into the evening repeating the experiment and saying nothing to his assistants. For the next seven weeks he worked at night in his laboratory experimenting alone and passing rays through various objects and blocking them with others. During this time he was the first in the world to see the bones of his own hand. It wasn't until 22 December that he told his wife of his discovery. He exposed her left hand to the rays for fifteen minutes and produced the first radiograph in the world, the left hand of Frau Roentgen showing the bones and her wedding ring.

Six days later, on 28th December 1895, a preliminary report was published in the *Proceedings of the Physico-Medical Society of Wurzburg*. Roentgen referred to his discovery as 'a new kind of light', and struggling for a name called them X-rays. (They are sometimes referred to as Roentgen rays and radiologists in the United States of America are sometimes referred to as roentgenologists.) He sent copies of his paper along with the radiograph to the leading scientists of the time, including Lord Kelvin and Arthur Schuster in Britain. Neither of them took any action at the time.

One scientist, Ernest Lechner, mentioned the discovery to his father, the editor of a Viennese newspaper, and on Sunday 5th January 1896 the news was published. A British reporter sent the news to London and the *Chronicle* and *Standard* reported the discovery of 'a new photography'. On 31st January the discovery was published in *Science* magazine. On 9th March 1896 Roentgen published a second paper 'Further observations on the properties of the X-ray', and on 3rd March 1897 a third paper was published. No further papers were published by Roentgen on X-rays.

Roentgen became the Director of the Physical Institute in Munich. In 1901 he received the first ever Nobel prize for Physics. The honour was soured by Lenard who demanded credit for the discovery. In fact both names had been submitted for consideration but the Academy chose to award the prize to Roentgen alone. The Royal Society awarded its Rumford medal in 1896 jointly to Lenard and Roentgen and in February 1896 a demonstration in Dublin of the rays was announced as the new Lenard or Roentgen rays.

Lenard was further distressed when the rays became universally known as Roentgen rays and didn't refrain from belittling Roentgen's achievement. In fact many scientists had generated X-rays without realizing their significance, William Crookes and J.J. Thomson in England and Arthur Willis Goodspeed in America. It is interesting that Crookes accused his suppliers of giving him faulty films which when he tried to use them were fogged in his laboratory. He had of course been generating X-rays.

The general public didn't appreciate the significance of X-rays and indeed the *Pall Mall Gazette* wrote in 1896, 'We are sick of the Roentgen rays. You can see other people's bones with the naked eye. On the revolting nature of this there is no need to dwell.' It was suggested they should be banned. Edward VII when Prince of Wales was shown the radiograph of a hand and exclaimed 'how disgusting'. The public thought the rays would be put to the wrong use and a clothing firm advertised the sale of X-ray proof underclothing for ladies. If they were really X-ray proof I hesitate to think how heavy and uncomfortable they would have been.

It is said Roentgen's work laid the foundation of atomic physics. Shortly after his discovery Antoine Henri Becquerel heard a lecture at the French Academy of Sciences on the subject. Becquerel put some uranium rocks in a drawer waiting to use them later. In the drawer were some photographic plates. On 1st March 1896 he opened the drawer to find that the plates showed an image of the rocks. He had discovered natural radioactivity. Also in 1896 Pierre and Marie Curie decided to pursue Becquerel's work and isolated Polonium and Radium. Along with Becquerel they shared the Nobel prize in 1903. (When my wife, Nancy, and I met when we were sixteen our first date was to the cinema where we saw Greer Garson and Walter Pidgeon in the film *Marie Curie*, the history of the work of the Curies in isolating radium. We have a print in our home of Pierre and Marie which depicts this discovery.)

It is remarkable to us today how quickly the discovery of X-rays was put to medical use. There were no ethical committees or bureaucratic regulations to delay progress. However nobody was aware of the side effects of this momentous discovery. As early as 7th January 1896, an electrician, Alan Archibald Swinton, made the first intentional radiograph and on January 13th 1896 took the first medical radiograph in the British Isles, an X-ray of his hand. Swinton grew up on the family estate in Berwickshire and boasted he had never passed an examination since the age of seventeen. He established the first X-ray laboratory in the British Isles at 66 Victoria Street, London. Lt-Colonel James Gifford gave the earliest demonstration of X-rays in London to the Royal Photographic Society at 12 Hanover Square. He was a well-to-do lacemaker. In those earliest days X-rays were mainly the province of physicists, electricians, photographers and other scientists. X-rays even made their way into the church when a congregational minister in Norfolk, the Rev. Frederick Walter, took an X-ray 'photograph' with an exposure time of thirty minutes. Although a very long exposure time it was shorter than his sermons!

The first X-ray taken at St Mary's Hospital was by the theatre instrument technician. The *Lancet* was the first medical journal in English to comment on X-rays. At first it made little of them, but a week later, having seen Swinton's hand, wrote that the discovery 'may be an aid to medical and surgical practice'. Professor Schuster wrote in the British Medical Journal that a most important discovery had been made. Sidney Rowlands, a 24-year-old medical student at St Bartholomew's Hospital, was asked by the BMJ to report on the medical applications of X-rays. On 24th February 1896 he demonstrated X-rays to the Medical Society of London and became the editor of the first radiological journal *Archives of Skiagraphy*. On 30th March 1896, Silvanus Thompson, a professor of physics and a highly respected academic, spoke to a medical audience and convinced them of the value of X-rays to the profession and urged them to form a Roentgen Society, which they duly did. In 1892 Dr John Macintyre held the position of medical electrician in addition to being surgeon in charge of the Nose and Throat Department of the Glasgow Royal Infirmary. In 1896 he was appointed Radiologist to the Glasgow Royal Infirmary, and his X-ray laboratory, as it was then called, was one of the first hospital X-ray departments in the world and thought by the Scots to be the first ever in the British Isles. Such was the speed at which hospitals developed the use of X-rays that it is difficult to confirm which was indeed the first hospital X-ray department. X-ray departments were set up in London hospitals between February and June 1896. The first in England is claimed to be at the Miller Hospital in Greenwich, established by Thomas Moore, the senior surgeon to the hospital. Moore became the first Treasurer of the Roentgen Society. X-rays were introduced to the London Hospital by Dr W.S. Hedley, a retired army medical officer. X-rays were used in St Bartholomew's Hospital early in 1896 and used to treat skin diseases before the end of 1896. At St Thomas's Hospital, Mr Stanley Kent gave a lecture to the Physical Society on 13 February calling it a new photography. Dr Barry Blacker who was their first radiologist also became the first British X-ray martyr.

Of special interest is the doctor who introduced X-rays to the Royal Free Hospital. This was Dr Florence Stoney, the first ever woman radiologist. Dr Florence Stoney came from a gifted Dublin family, both her father and brother were Fellows of the Royal College of Surgeons in Ireland. Students still compete for the Stoney Memorial Gold Medal at the College. Women were not admitted to study medicine at Dublin University, so Florence Stoney entered the London School of Medicine for Women. She qualified with honours and obtained her MD in 1898. In 1902 she specialized in radiology. During the First World War, against heavy opposition, she led a medical corps consisting entirely of women to Belgium. They established a 135-bedded hospital which after heavy bombing moved to a chateau near Cherbourg. To power the X-ray apparatus and light the hospital they adapted a water wheel in the grounds. In 1915 Florence Stoney was given a full time commission by the War Office in charge of the X-ray department of a 1000 bedded hospital in Fulham. She was the first woman doctor to be given such a post.

Burrows in his excellent book says the greatest of the British pioneers in radiology was Dr Alfred Earnest Barclay and refers to him as 'the grand old man of British Radiology'. Barclay was introduced to radiology at the breakfast table. His father reading the *Manchester Guardian* said 'a man claims to have discovered a new kind of light that will penetrate solids and show the bones of the hand – how absurd.'

Following the earliest days of radiology when X-rays were used only to locate foreign bodies and bone fractures their use spread rapidly to other areas such as the detection of kidney stones, and the investigation of bone and joint disease. H. Strauss in Berlin as early as 1896 used gelatine capsules filled with iron oxide and bismuth to visualize the digestive tract. In 1897 Dr W.B. Cannon in Harvard observed the movements of the stomach of a cat using bismuth. In 1898 Lewis Jones FRCP in St Bartholomew's Hospital said that apart from X-raying foreign bodies and bone fractures, the use of X-rays will make it possible to diagnose lung tuberculosis earlier than one could with a stethoscope.

How true that proved to be. Soon after 1895 workers tried contrast agents (dyes) to show the vascular system (blood vessels) in animals and human cadavers. Examples of the vascular system were studied in the dead foetus in 1899 with the injection of four pounds of mercury. The exposure time was twenty minutes. This may have been an enormous benefit for the knowledge and development of investigations for blood vessel diseases but I could imagine a great outcry against such investigations if carried out today.

Barclay was before his time in many areas and in 1909 read a paper before the Roentgen Society, 'The value of X-rays in Diseases of the Digestive Tract'. He later published a book on *The Oesophagus and Stomach*. It was in 1910 that barium was first used for the gastrointestinal tract. In 1915 thorium was used for certain examinations of the kidney (retrograde pyelography), and thorotrast in the 1920s. In 1924 Graham and Cole introduced contrast (dye) investigations of the gall bladder. In 1927 Moniz in Portugal first performed a cerebral arteriogram (the injection of contrast into the major arteries to the head for the investigation of brain disorders). In 1929 Dos Santos, Lamas and Caldas in Lisbon reported the first percutaneous lumbar aortogram (the injection into the main blood vessel in the abdomen through a long needle introduced through the back). This was a major step in the investigation of blood vessel disorders in the abdomen, pelvis and legs. In 1929 uroselectan was first used for the intravenous examination of the renal tract (the kidneys, ureters and bladder). Over the years and especially since the Second World War refinement after refinement of contrast media has led to the development of safer and more sophisticated tri-iodinated compounds, both high and low osmolar, ionic and non-ionic to examine every organ and every blood vessel in the body. In 1953 Seldinger introduced percutaneous catheterization (the passing of catheters into the major blood vessels). This opened another chapter in radiological investigation and treatment.

The first military X-ray apparatus was introduced into the Royal Victoria Military Hospital in Netley as early as 1896. This was due to Surgeon General William Flack Stevenson, an Irishman who qualified in Dublin in 1844. In 1895 he held the rank of Lt-Colonel and was Professor of Clinical and Military Medicine in the Royal Army Medical School. The first military casualties to be X-rayed were during the Abyssinian War of 1896 in the military hospital in Naples. In 1898

Surgeon-Major W.C. Beevor wrote 'I maintain that it is now the duty of every civilized nation to supply its wounded with an X-ray apparatus.' He was the first to use X-rays in the field of battle. He purchased a portable X-ray apparatus himself. X-rays were used in the Sudan War of 1898 by Surgeon-Major Battersby, another Irishman. A fixed bicycle ridden by army volunteers was used to charge the batteries to produce the X-rays.

Soon after the discovery of X-rays as well as their diagnostic use they were used to treat all manners of disease. Their use in the treatment of malignant disease has greatly influenced the outcome of many cancers, and radiotherapy departments are found in many centres throughout the world. However the X-rays that can cure can sometimes harm and this was not appreciated immediately on their discovery. It was just three months after Roentgen's discovery that reports appeared of the harmful effects of X-rays. These included, erythema, radiation burns, radiation dermatitis, radiation ulcers, bone necrosis and cancers. The early pioneers suffered and there were many finger and upper limb amputations. There were many deaths. In 1936 a martyrs' memorial was erected in Hamburg which included 169 names, 14 of them British. It appears not all are included however.

I have concentrated on the early days in the development of X-rays mainly in the first half of the twentieth century. However following the Second World War in the second half of the twentieth century even more amazing developments were to occur, beyond the imagination of even the most educated and informed of the medical profession. Ultrasound developed from the echo sounding used to detect submarines during the war. The great pioneer in the British Isles was Professor Ian Donald in Glasgow. It is said that ultrasound now makes up about 40% of patient imaging. Medical specialists in isotope imaging appeared in the late 1960s. A positron brain scan which can detect function was performed in 1964. Positron Emission Tomography revealing anatomy and function is a technique of the 1990s. However it was image intensification in the 1960s that took radiology screening out of the dark, giving excellent visualization in the light that paved the way to practical procedures of ever increasing complexity for diagnosis and treatment. This has led to Interventional Radiology, now a growing specialty within radiology, the use of which in many cases avoids major surgical incisions for the treatment of patients. Computed Tomography

(CT) invented by Godfrey Hounsfield and clinically developed by Dr James Ambrose in Atkinson Morley's hospital was introduced in 1972. It is said by some to be the most important radiological development since the discovery of X-rays. Cross sectional visualization, including three dimensional imaging of anatomy and diseased tissues reached a new sophistication leading to improved diagnostic capabilities. These techniques were further improved with the introduction of Magnetic Resonance Imaging (MRI).

Interventional Radiology owes much to Dotter in the United States of America who in 1964 introduced percutaneous angioplasty (the introduction of balloons through the skin to dilate narrowed arteries).

Today radiology is in the forefront of patient management in both diagnosis and treatment and the discovery of this radiant light has come a long way since that Friday night on 8th November 1895.

CHAPTER 4

The Royal College of Radiologists

THE ESTABLISHMENT OF THE Royal College of Radiologists was due to the amalgamation of many societies over the years from 1897 to 1975 and was one of repeated change.

The story begins only eighteen months after Roentgen's discovery of X-rays. On June 31st 1897 the Roentgen Society was formed following the suggestion of Professor Silvanus Thompson to a group of doctors. At its inception there were more scientists in the society than doctors and soon the medical profession wished for its own radiological society and in 1902 formed the Electrotherapeutic Society, radiologists being involved in both the diagnostic and therapeutic properties of X-rays. This society became part of the Royal Society of Medicine in 1905.

The Roentgen Society remained and in 1917 joined the Electrotherapeutic Society to form the British Association for the Advancement of Radiology and Physiotherapy.

Today it is difficult to understand why physiotherapy should have been associated with radiology, but the union was fragile and didn't last long. Perhaps it had its origin in the use of electricity in treatments by physiotherapists. However further union in 1924 led to a major change, the formation of the British Institute of Radiology (BIR) which exists to this day and consists of radiologists, radiographers (X-ray technicians), scientists and many involved in the commercial world of radiological equipment and drugs. The British Institute of Radiology obtained a Royal Charter in 1958 and the patronage of the Queen in 1979. This institute is a forum for discussion between all disciplines involved in the science of radiology: it is concerned with organizing lectures and seminars but has no role in the examination or certification in medical radiology. From its earliest years courses were given at the BIR and the first diploma for radiologists was the Diploma of Radiology and Electrology (DMRE), granted by examination by the University of Cambridge. This was a test for both diagnostic and therapeutic radiology.

In 1930 diagnostic and therapeutic radiology were recognized as different subjects and two diplomas were created, the DMRD in diagnosis and the DMRT in radiotherapy. In 1934 the British Association of Radiology was formed purely for diagnostic radiologists and Dr James Brailsford was elected its first president. The following year a surgeon, George Stebbings, formed the Society of Radiotherapists for those interested in the radiotherapy treatment of cancer.

On February 17th 1939 both of these societies united to form the Faculty of Radiologists, with the two sections having equal representation on the council of the Faculty. The first annual meeting was in June 1939 in Liverpool and Dr R.E. Roberts of Liverpool was elected the first President. For four years the administrative office was in 32 Welbeck Street, the home of the BIR, but in 1943 the Faculty moved to the Royal College of Surgeons in Lincoln's Inn Fields. Dr Rohan Williams of St Mary's Hospital, Paddington, London when Honorary Secretary of the Faculty in 1953, later Warden and then President in 1961, said that the Faculty should aim for College status and a Royal Charter. The main thrust to form a college was initiated by Dr James Bull, a neuroradiologist of international status, in the years 1969 to 1972, when he was President of the Faculty. The College, consisting of the two faculties of diagnostic radiology and radiotherapy, was formed during the Presidency of Howard Middlemiss, who became its first President in 1975. The Royal Charter was granted the same year. An appeal for premises was conducted under the chairmanship of Lord Robens and in 1976, 38 Portland Place, London was purchased by The Charles Wolfson Trust for the College, which purchased the house from the Trust in 1979. On December 19th 1979, the Duke of Edinburgh officially opened the College during the Presidency of Professor Robert Steiner, who admitted the Duke as an Honorary Fellow.

The College objectives are:

The advancement of the science and practice of radiology.

The furtherance of public education.

The promotion of study and research.

The College is responsible for the setting of professional standards of practice in Clinical Radiology and Clinical Oncology, which are its two Faculties. The College acts as a major provider of education in both clinical radiology and clinical oncology through lectures and conferences. It accredits hospital departments for training in both disciplines. It conducts examinations for the Fellowship of the College which is a recommendation for consultant posts in both disciplines in the National Health Service. It publishes scientific journals, reports and guidance. It liaises with government, other medical Royal Colleges, Associations and Institutes.

A great deal of my life has been involved with the Royal College of Radiologists, of which I was Registrar from 1981 to 1985, Vice-President from 1985 to 1987 and President from 1989 to 1992. All my years with the College have been happy and fulfilling.

Various medical men have influenced the progress of my career leading to me holding academic posts in the College, clinical posts in the National Health Service, principally in St Mary's Hospital, Paddington, and in St Mary's Hospital Medical School.

Having spent three months as a general duties medical officer on an Air Force station I was summoned to see the senior surgeon in the RAF. This was Air Commodore Dixon who later was Air Vice Marshal Sir Peter Dixon, affectionately known as 'Dickie'. It was he who started my future career. He seemed, for all my time in the RAF, to be concerned for my welfare, and many times tried to persuade me to make my future career as a surgeon in the RAF. He posted me to the RAF hospital in Ely, Cambridgeshire to work under Wing Commander, later Air Commodore, Malcolm who was a good surgical teacher. I learnt much from both men and it was due to them that I obtained my Fellowship in surgery without which the steps that followed would never have happened. I remember them both with affection.

The doctors mentioned as instrumental in the development of the college also had an influence on my life.

Perhaps the next great influence was Dr Rohan Williams, Consultant Radiologist and Director of the Department of Radiology, St Mary's Hospital, Paddington, London. In 1957 the number of applications for trainee posts in radiology was enormous, often as many as eighty for each. I had the added disadvantage that my medical school had been in Dublin, whereas almost all the applicants came from this side of the Irish Channel, and indeed many were from London teaching hospitals. I was short-listed along with seven other doctors and one was from St Mary's Hospital and had an unpaid post in the Department of Radiology.

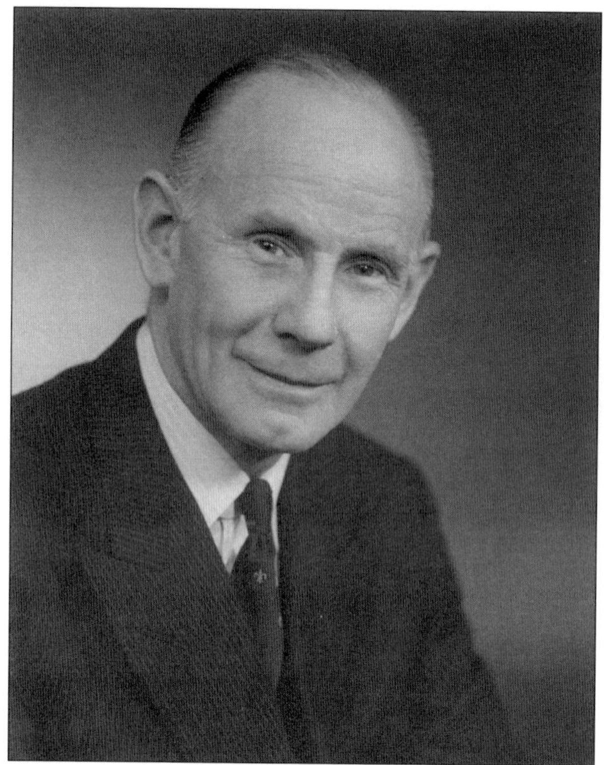

Dr Rohan Williams. Past Director, Dept. of Radiology, St Mary's Hospital, Paddington. Past President Faculty of Radiology

Although many had higher qualifications in medicine I was the only one with a Fellowship in surgery. It was very debatable whether or not this was any advantage over the equivalent degree in medicine. To my delight and surprise Rohan must have favoured me as the committee appointed me to the post and it is due to him that my career in radiology started. Throughout the time I worked under Rohan Williams he gave me support and encouragement and what I believe was friendship despite the difference in our medical status at the time. Rohan taught me my basic radiology. Moreover his personal qualities and behaviour were an example of how to conduct myself if and when appointed as a consultant. He was one of the most conscientious doctors I've ever known and the essence of academic honesty and integrity. Rohan was tall, slim, immaculate in dress, obsessional in work and play and always smoking a cigarette. He was an excellent teacher, patient and caring. I've never known any doctor agonize more on making an error.

His loyalty to St Mary's Hospital and its medical school was etched on his heart. He accompanied the first rugby XV team at the weekends and acted as touch judge. He was popular with his juniors and his colleagues who gave him unqualified respect. His skill and expertise in radiology was acknowledged internationally. Rohan was educated at Epsom College and read medicine at St Mary's Hospital Medical School, London University. He was a Cheadle gold medallist in 1929.

He held many Fellowships of the medical Royal Colleges and an Honorary Fellowship was awarded to him from the Australasian College of Radiologists in 1960 and the Faculty of Radiology in Ireland in 1962. He was President of the British Institute of Radiology in 1944 and Warden of the Faculty of Radiologists in 1956 to 1961 when he was appointed President. It was while he was President I obtained my Fellowship of the Faculty by examination and Rohan launched me on my speaking career by inviting me to give the address at the graduates Fellowship dinner. He encouraged me in my early clinical research and we published a paper together on lung changes during thoracic operations. I read that paper at the Royal College of Surgeons and my lecture career began.

Rohan was Hunterian Professor of the Royal College of Surgeons in 1955. It was Rohan's wish for the Faculty to achieve College status which it did in 1975, but sadly he never lived to see this.

In 1963, Rohan came to me in the department. 'Oscar, I'd like you to show some visitors around the hospital. I don't feel up to doing it, as I've just discovered I've a cancer of my lung.'

'My God, are you sure, sir?'

'Yes, there's no doubt.'

I was devastated as this man meant much to me and had nurtured me. His heavy smoking had caught up with him. Rohan died on 17th March 1963, St Patrick's day, while he was still President of the Faculty. His Presidency was taken by Dr Thomas Lodge, later Sir Thomas Lodge, and I was appointed consultant into the vacant post at St Mary's Hospital

I missed Rohan enormously and have described the feeling as being like a one-legged man without a crutch. He is another man whom I remember with great affection and I owe him much for any success I have subsequently had.

I first met Dr James Bull, who spearheaded the establishment of the Royal College of Radiologists, when he sat on the appointments committee for the consultant post I obtained at St Mary's Hospital in 1963. I was to become friendly with him in later years. James was an imposing man, slim in build, handsome, immaculately dressed, distinguished in appearance and serious in demeanour. He was the epitome of an English gentleman in style and manners. His sense of humour however was not obvious. He was educated in Repton and read medicine at Gonville and Caius, Cambridge and St George's Hospital Medical School. From 1940 to 1946 he held the rank of Major in the Royal Army Medical Corps. He had a difficult war.

Posted to Singapore, he was called to the top floor of the hospital just before the Japanese Army entered it, killing all doctors, nurses and patients on the ground floor which he had just left. James was captured and spent the remainder of the war in Changi prisoner of war camp. This was the fate of a number of doctors who became colleagues later, Brian Mayne, Bill Young, Bill Frankland and others I knew less well than these.

James Bull after the war specialized in neuroradiology, wrote extensively and lectured widely. He was consultant in the National Hospital for Nervous Diseases, Queens Square, Maida Vale Hospital for Nervous Diseases and St George's Hospital, Hyde Park Corner, London. He became Consultant Adviser in Diagnostic Radiology to the Department of Health and Consultant Neuroradiologist to the Royal Navy. He held numerous distinguished academic posts, Dean of the Institute of Neurology, President of the British Institute of Radiology in 1960, President of the Section of Radiology of the Royal Society of Medicine 1968–1969 and President of the Faculty of Radiologists from 1969 to 1972. He was President of the European Society of Neuroradiologists from 1972 to 1975. James was awarded an Honorary Fellowship of the Royal Society of Medicine and of the American College of Radiologists.

James and I became close friends when I lectured in Radiological Anatomy at King's College, University of London. The pre-clinical students came from King's College Hospital, Westminster Hospital and St George's Hospital Medical Schools.

My aim in these lectures was not to teach radiology but by using radiological imaging to stress the clinical importance of anatomy and stimulate this interest by showing examples of disease involving anatomical regions. James Bull felt passionately that anatomy should be

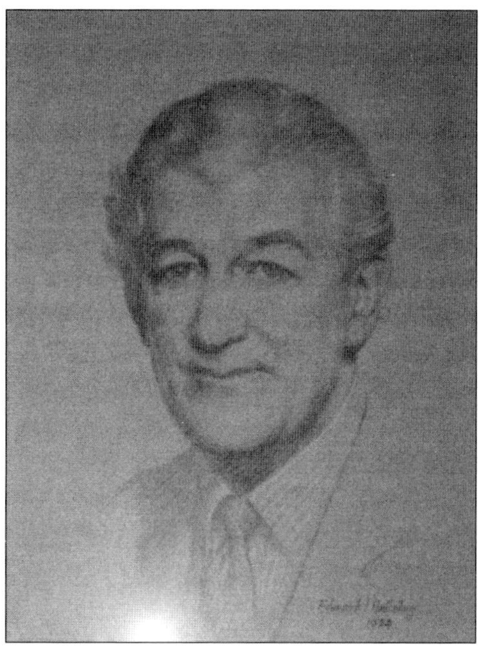

Dr James Bull. Consultant Neuro-Radiologist, Queens Square, London. Past President Faculty of Radiologists

taught by clinical radiologists and strived to encourage medical schools to this end. He came to King's College to hear me lecture. His opinion of my work was very complimentary and he wrote an article on this manner of teaching for the *British Medical Journal* and delivered a lecture on his thesis at the Royal College of Physicians, mentioning my lectures and their effect. James Bull's contribution to radiology and indeed medicine and teaching earned great respect in the United Kingdom and internationally.

Our friendship came late in his career and was cut short for me when James was killed in a car accident.

Sir Howard Middlemiss was one of the most colourful men among the radiologists I've known. He was medium in height, stocky in build, sported a van Dyke beard, and had a smiling face with lively penetrating eyes which never left you as he spoke.

Howard had an ebullient manner, graced by a sparkling sense of humour. He spoke quietly and rapidly with a staccato rhythm but holding your attention whatever the subject. I admired him for his engaging personality and his outstanding contribution to radiology. It was said of Howard that he could enter a revolving door behind you but come out first. Such was his drive and determination.

Howard was born in Northumbria, educated in Repton and qualified in medicine in Durham University. He joined the Royal Army Medical Corps after qualification and served in Normandy and India. He specialized in clinical radiology and in 1949 was appointed Director of Radiology in Bristol. He had a flair for administration and was a natural leader. He built a reputation for his department in Bristol for its clinical work and teaching. He attracted the best young radiologists to Bristol and was enthusiastic in encouraging them to achieve clinical and academic success. In 1966 he was awarded a personal chair in Bristol University. He served in the university as Dean of the Faculty of Medicine from 1977 to 1980.

Perhaps Howard's greatest achievement was to travel to developing countries to teach radiology and to establish departments of radiology which he helped to equip and staff. Howard had a hand in promoting a Basic Radiology System supplied by the World Health Organization (WHO). Even in 1983 when the first of these machines was supplied the WHO wrote that 70% of the world's population, most of them living in developing countries, couldn't get an X-ray examination. X-ray equipment and spare parts were too complex and expensive. Philips Medical Systems produced this simple X-ray machine capable of working on batteries as well as standard single phase mains supply. The machines and training manuals were clinically tested in 21 countries before the end of 1985. Apart from very minor problems all clinical test reports were favourable.

Professor Middlemiss sent young radiologists to many places in Africa, West Indies, Malaysia and Burma. He encouraged radiologists and radiographers to come to England for further study. For his work overseas he was awarded the Companionship of the Order of St Michael and St George (CMG). Howard was Adviser in Radiology to the governments of Burma, Iran, Laos, Malaysia, Nigeria, Turkey, Uganda, Phillipines, South Vietnam, Tanzania and numerous universities abroad from 1953 to 1980. He was a Fellow of the major Medical Royal Colleges, an Honorary Member of the Radiological Society of North America (RSNA), the Swedish Radiological Society and an Honorary Member of the Royal Australasian College of Radiologists. He lectured extensively and gave a large number of eponymous lectures

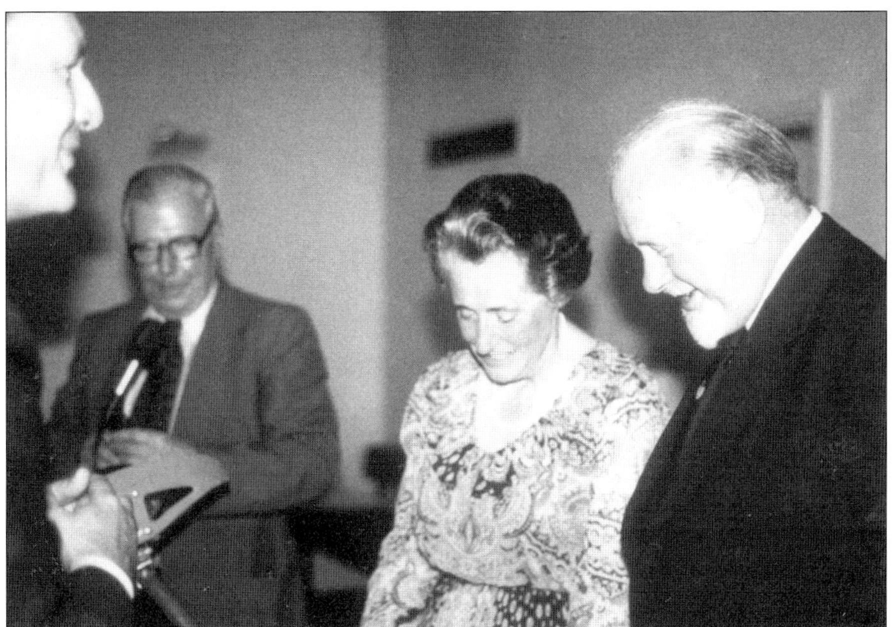

Sir Howard Middlemiss. Professor of Radiology Bristol University, Past President Royal College of Radiologists, and Lady Middlemiss. Dr Frank Ross, Consultant Radiologist Bristol Royal Infirmary, on left

at home and abroad. He was instrumental in establishing the Royal College of Radiologists following the initiative of James Bull and was the first President of the Royal College of Radiologists in 1975. Howard was knighted in 1981 for his contribution to Radiology and in 1982 awarded the Gold Medal of the Royal College of Radiologists.

Howard and I were members of the Shadows Radiological Visiting Club and despite two mishaps our friendship survived. He was very senior to me and when I was young and inexperienced, long before getting a consultant post or being invited to join the Shadows, I was asked to review a book he wrote, and my review was less than complimentary. Friends telephoned me to tell me I had committed medical suicide. I would have trouble getting a consultant post, especially in the south of England. Howard in all our subsequent years as friends has never mentioned this. When, years later, I was a relatively young consultant at St Mary's Hospital, Howard asked me if I would go for the British Council to lecture in Ghana for six weeks. I agreed and spent months in preparing lectures and hundreds of slides. I checked with Ghana the best time to go and was given the date, and the name of the hotel in which I was to stay. Nancy was going to join me for the last month.

When I got off the plane in Accra, my body was hit by a blast of heat like I'd never felt before. I felt like a large plank of wood had hit me, sapping all my energy. So this was Africa. I expected to be met by some medical representatives of the hospital, but was surprised that only a driver waited for me. He said I would get through the airport much quicker if I put some money into my passport when I showed it. I thought it unwise to try bribery on my first visit to Africa and so it took a long time to get clear and out to the waiting car. There was another African waiting by the car. I have never found out who these two people were but I think they worked in a hospital store. They informed me that arrangements had changed and they were to take me to a room in the University campus some miles from Accra and miles from the hospital in which I was to lecture. This seemed strange, but they seemed to know all about me and my visit. When we arrived at the University campus I was shown to a room furnished with a bed, a table and a chair. It was lit by a naked light bulb. They then left telling me I would be collected next morning. It was eight o'clock and dark and I was hungry. I was surprised and alarmed to see a guard outside my door, an African over six foot tall carrying a machete. I didn't know if he was there to keep me in or others out. The drivers had pointed out a cafe across the road from my room. I decided to go there but found a man locking it up. I persuaded him to let me have a bottle of coca-cola. Back in the room I realized I hadn't got a bottle opener. I asked the guard if he could open it and to my surprise he bit off the tin top. Unfortunately there was an epidemic of cholera in Ghana at the time and it was impossible to drink from it. Even if there hadn't been cholera my sensitivity is such that I wouldn't have drunk it. I was tired, lonely, confused and anxious. When I decided to go to bed I couldn't get into it. After much fiddling I realized it was made up in such a way to avoid snakes getting between the sheets. There were plenty of large lizards around the building which didn't bother me, but you had to make sure none got into the room. Apparently they could drop onto the bed from the ceiling.

The room was air conditioned but it was a primitive system and made a noise the whole night. The following morning the same car arrived and took me to the hospital. I was shown to a similar room, similarly furnished and left. No member of the medical staff came to see me. I spent some time revising my lectures. Exasperated I went in search of the Professor of Medicine. I found him eventually. He seemed surprised to see me and seemed to have forgotten I was coming to Ghana. I asked him about the lectures and he told me the students were all doing examinations and then going on holiday. I could hardly believe what he was saying and indeed what was happening. At about five o'clock I was returned to my room in the university campus. I went across to the cafe to get a meal and found it empty, apart from a white girl sitting at a table. I was amazed and pleased as here was someone I could talk to. I joined her.

'Where are you from?'

'America.'

'What are you doing here?'

'I'm estimating the growth rate of the African sparrow.'

'You are – –what?'

'Estimating the growth rate of the African sparrow.'

'Why are you doing that?'

'I'm an ornithologist.'

'Really. Where do you do this estimation?'

'I've been working on this for some months in a laboratory on the campus, but I leave to-morrow.'

I couldn't believe all this was happening and since leaving England my mind hadn't been working normally. Since arriving in Ghana the sequence of events seemed surreal.

'Are you doing your experiments tonight?'

'Yes.'

'Well, I'm a doctor and am going to ask you a favour. Before you answer, I want to tell you that I'm normal and safe in every way. Can I come with you tonight?'

She looked hard at me and after a measurable pause said 'Yes.'

She drove me in a battered Volkswagen Beetle to the laboratory. We were the only people in the building.

There she went to a cage where there were birds caught for her in the wild. She took one out and placed it in a beaker, weighing the beaker and bird. She passed oxygen into the beaker and measured the oxygen consumption of the bird over a given length of time. She killed the bird and weighed it. I couldn't watch her wringing the neck of the bird. When shown what to do I helped by timing the oxygen input and measuring the oxygen consumed on a primitive measuring device, noting down the figures. She did innumerable calculations but I'm unaware as to how she reached her eventual conclusions. At this stage I wondered what in the name of heaven I was doing, having come to Africa to lecture to medical students, the only work I'd done and was likely to do was to help estimate the growth rate of the African sparrow.

She took me back to my guarded room. I asked her to send me a copy of her completed paper to London. I never saw her again.

The next day the car arrived to take me to the hospital. I asked to meet the hospital consultant in radiology. He wasn't interested in me and didn't know what to do with me. That afternoon he took me to his house where he played classical music on a gramophone as we sat in his lounge. I began to think all this was a nightmare. I offered to do a case for him the next day but when I got to the hospital he said the patient had been discharged. My thoughts were in turmoil and I decided to phone home to tell Nancy not to come and discuss with her my resolve to leave Ghana as soon as possible. I couldn't do this as the telephones were not operating because of a strike.

I went to the Professor of Medicine again.

'What can I do for you?' he asked.

'Firstly, get me out of that guarded room on the University campus. Secondly, get me a seat on the first plane to leave Ghana.'

He showed no sign of surprise.

'Stay in my house tonight. We're having a party you might like to join.'

'Thank you, I will.'

The next day I was taken to the airport by the Professor.

As I boarded the plane he said, 'There is one thing we can't understand. Why are you so keen to work?'

I smiled but didn't reply.

Back in London, I telephoned Howard and went to Bristol to see him. I told him my story and he listened carefully.

'Oscar, in Africa, you have to wait a long time to move a centimetre.'

'Howard, I'm the wrong man for this. I haven't the patience or the stamina to put up with that.'

I reported my saga to the British Council who came over to lunch at St Mary's to talk about it. They seemed less concerned than I thought they should be. As they were leaving they asked, 'When would you be willing to go back?'

'Never.'

Six months after I arrived home the ornithologist girl's paper on the growth rate of the African sparrow arrived. I wasn't surprised not to be mentioned as a co-author, but disappointed I didn't appear in the acknowledgements!

Howard and I met frequently in subsequent years but he never referred to the African visit that was a disappointment for both of us. On 27th April 1983 Howard died at the early age of sixty seven. His contribution to radiology internationally was unique.

Chapter 5

College Commitments

My first involvement in the committees of the Royal College of Radiologists was when I was elected a member of the Education Committee. Unfortunately this met on a Friday afternoon at 2.00 p.m., and I lectured at King's College in the Strand on Radiological Anatomy at 2.00 p.m. on Fridays. I was torn between two duties. I argued to myself that with regard to medical education it was perhaps better to be doing it than talking about it, so I continued to give the lectures. I rushed from the Strand to the College in Portland Place at 3.00 p.m., but invariably too late to make any contribution. John Laws was the Warden of the College at the time and chaired the committee. I was surprised when later he supported me to become the Registrar of the College. I think he knew how important these lectures were to me and indeed to the students. They packed into the lecture theatre and even sat on the stairways as the benches were full.

We had some major problems when I was Registrar and it is fortunate that John and I had a deep and mutual friendship which enabled us to tackle them as with one voice.

The most engaging and significant problem concerned the managerial control of Departments of Radiology throughout the United Kingdom. Radiographers, i.e., the X-ray technicians who operated the apparatus, belonged to the Society of Radiographers and the College of Radiographers. Both of these bodies moved strongly for the day-to-day management of departments to be in the control of radiographers. They worked in departments full time whereas radiologists often divided their time between different hospitals or had a few sessions in private consulting rooms. Each department had a superintendent radiographer, responsible for the radiographers, for their duties and quality of work, but the departments were managed by the radiologist. The budget for the department, which was sizeable, was held by the radiologist. By and large throughout the United Kingdom, the relationship between the radiographers and radiologists was good. There was mutual respect and the excellence of the radiographers and their contribution to the care of the patients couldn't be overestimated. However for whatever reason, perhaps power and finance, the College of Radiographers moved to have control of the department budget and the day to day management. They were following an example set by some departments of biochemistry where laboratory technicians had been given managerial control. I felt strongly that the decision-making in management in a clinical department must remain in the hands of medically qualified personnel, in this case the radiologist. Such a physician should hold the budget and be responsible for the spending of that budget in consultation with the other departmental physicians. The size of the budget and the use of it were related to the other needs of the hospital and discussed with the medical committee to which the radiographers hadn't access. It was of course important that the superintendant radiographer's views should be part of the consultation process.

The Royal College of Radiologists had for years had liaison meetings with the College of Radiographers and during these difficult years the College of Radiographers raised the subject of managerial control at every meeting. The atmosphere at these meetings was cold and almost hostile. The most hostile of the radiographers were male. At one particular meeting I didn't help the atmosphere when I said, 'I've great respect for the work of the radiographers without which we cannot function, but I will not move one centimetre to allow radiographers to have managerial control of clinical departments of radiology.'

I thought it necessary to have this opinion stated firmly and to make sure all knew where we stood and indeed what was the view of the Royal College of Radiologists.

There was a hush in the room and one radiographer, a male, said, 'Dr Craig, would you repeat that please.'

'I certainly will.'

When I repeated it he said, 'I think it important that we minute this carefully so that the position of the Royal College of Radiologists is clear. I want it known how open your college is to discussion!'

'Yes, do that please.'

To this day I regret it was necessary to have this battle. Radiographers do a marvellous job and thankfully the relationships between the radiographers and the radiologists remained cordial in the hospitals. However the atmosphere at the College level remained unsettled. It had reached a stage where it was necessary to ask for an opinion from the

Chief Medical Officer on behalf of the Department of Health. It was ruled that the management of Departments of Radiology and the budgets must remain in the hands of a medically qualified person i.e. the radiologist.

I wasn't popular with the College of Radiographers.

In recent years the work of the radiographers has changed considerably and selected radiographers perform more complex tasks and their skills are considerable. Their technical work in Computed Tomography (CT) and Magnetic Resonance Imaging (MRI) is considerable and their involvement in breast screening is essential in running the service. However at the end of the day the outcome of radiological examinations requires medical judgement, the results require a medical opinion, and the interventional techniques now performed in departments of radiology require lengthy medical training and detailed knowledge of medical skills. To my knowledge the battle over managerial control of departments has not recurred.

It was the use of X-rays in the treatment of cancer that produced the union of the two disciplines in one college i.e. clinical radiology and clinical oncology. In recent years the treatment of cancer includes the use of cytotoxic drugs and doctors not skilled in the use of X-rays also treat cancers and are termed Medical Oncologists; their college is most often the Royal College of Physicians. I am in favour of a union of medical oncologists and clinical oncologists, most of whom are also Fellows of the Royal College of Physicians, into one academic body, and this could be within the Royal Colleges or even separately. This seems reasonable to me as both disciplines are concerned with the one goal, i.e. the treatment of cancer. At the present time they meet in a liaison committee.

I was elected President of the College in 1989, the term of office being three years. This was to be a very busy time in my life. I find it difficult to express the enormous thrill it gave me when I received the phone call from the college telling me the results of the voting. It is not expected that the vice-president would become the next president and indeed I hadn't held office in the college for the previous two years. The joy of all my family added to the excitement. I felt a surge of pride in holding the office of President. I felt this was the pinnacle of my career and that all the hard work, the good and especially the bad times had been worth it. Doctoring had always been the centre of my life but I never imagined I would ever hold the most prestigious post in my specialty. It was beyond my dreams. I was touched by the faith my colleagues had in me. If only they knew how my life had always been full of doubt about my ability. I've always thought I had a pedestrian mind with not much originality. Of course in the conduct of my professional life I had hidden these doubts. A failing from which I suffered was the love of 'centre stage'. Now I had it in a big way. Would I be successful? If ever it was time to shed doubt – it was now.

I had a regret that my mother and father weren't alive to share this moment. Their early sacrifices for my career would have been rewarded. My sister Maxime had died from Hodgkin's Disease and I wish too she could have joined our celebration.

The appointment came at the best possible time. I was Director of the Department of Radiology at St Mary's Hospital and had built up the consultant staff and re-equipped the department. It was possible for me to give my time to the college and the affairs of Clinical Radiology and Clinical Oncology within the NHS. I met with the managers of the hospital to explain that I would be attending to these medical duties for part of almost every day. The hospital would still be served fully by my colleagues in the department who were happy to fulfil any extra duties. I was fortunate with their co-operation and fortunate that the hospital also gave its blessing to my duties to the college. I even spoke to the government's Chief Medical Officer to clear my conscience of receiving a salary from the hospital while officiating as President of the college. He reassured me it was essential for the running of the NHS that time must be given to hold office in Medical Royal Colleges.

The number of committees I had to attend was daunting. I had to chair the Council of the College and the Annual General Meeting, and attend all the other committees ex officio. These committees included the Faculty Boards of Clinical Radiology and Clinical Oncology, the Education Committee and the Finance Committee. I chaired the liaison committee with the College of Radiographers each alternate meeting and attended the council meetings of the British Institute of Radiology to represent the college. During those three years I attended the hospital every morning and the college in the afternoon, gave my lectures, wrote for the journals and gave tutorials each week. I also attended the meetings of the Medical Protection Society and continued with my work in medico-legal medicine. I was busy and happy. I had an en suite bedroom in the college as well as my office, but in those three years I only slept in the college on one or two occasions. I preferred to go home at night and as I left very late the traffic was light and I drove home quickly. I was amazed at the number of official dinners I had to attend. As President of a Medical Royal College I was invited automatically to all medical college dinners and most medical dinners that were held by the Department of Health and medical and para-medical Societies. At times there were three or four a week. Nancy came to about half of them. It isn't surprising that my weight increased significantly. We had our own College dinners as well and I loved these and Nancy thoroughly enjoyed being the hostess. She took to it like a duck to water! We miss them still. I made many mistakes. I had to give a 'state of the college' address at each Annual Dinner and there were times when I spoke overlong. I can only put this down to over-enthusiasm. There was invariably a bet on some tables as to how long the speech would last.

I attended some crucial NHS committees to represent the college along with other College Presidents, the Standing Medical Advisory Committee, advisory to the Chief Medical Officer, and the Joint Consultants Committee, attended also by the Chief Medical Officer and members of the Department of Health. For a time I represented the college on the General Medical Council, I also attended the Council of the Royal College of Surgeons representing radiology for the three years of my presidency. This was most instructive and as a Fellow of the Royal College of Surgeons and a past surgeon I enjoyed this enormously. I thought this representation was well worth while but sadly it has ceased.

When I was President there was no separate representation of Northern Ireland in the Royal College of Radiologists so I formed a Standing Northern Ireland Committee and attended the first meeting in Belfast. There are Standing Committees for Wales and Scotland. The chairmen of these committees attend Council. A committee I thought extremely important to the profession was the Conference of Medical Royal Colleges and their Faculties. The committee consisted of the Presidents of the Colleges and Faculties from throughout the United Kingdom and presented to the Department of Health and the Secretary of State a consensus opinion on medical matters. The largest Colleges were the Royal College of Surgeons, represented by Terence English, the Royal College of Physicians represented by Margaret Turner-Warwick, the Royal College of Obstetricians and Gynaecologists by

George Pinker and then Stanley Simmons and the Royal College of General Practitioners, the largest of all, represented by Denis Periera Gray and Stuart Carne. Other colleges were smaller but had an equal voice. While I was President there were three Secretaries of State for Health. The first was Kenneth Clarke, the second William Waldegrave and the third Virginia Bottomley. Presidents of Medical Colleges are elected for varying reasons, because of their academic record, their international reputation or their overall popularity, but as individuals they are often politically naive. There are exceptions. At the end of one particular meeting Kenneth Clarke asked us not to talk to the press, but as we left the meeting to our surprise he was doing just that. The most popular of the three as Secretary of State was William Waldegrave. He entertained us to dinner in small groups to facilitate communication and get to know us better. We thought he listened to us and was willing to fight for our needs. We were all surprised but delighted. We were unfamiliar with such treatment from politicians. I said at the time, 'I doubt if he will last long in this post with these views.'

Too soon he was replaced by Virginia Bottomley. At a cocktail party given by the Department of Health Virginal Bottomley said to me, 'Dr Craig, what are the problems in your specialty?'

'I don't think we could discuss these fully at a cocktail party.'

'Try me.'

'Well, I'll start with manpower and then go on to equipment needs. We have the lowest figures for medical manpower in clinical radiology in the industrialized west of Europe. We are lower than France, Germany, Sweden, Denmark, Norway and others. I shall enlarge on this shortly but tell you that our equipment is on average over twenty years old i.e. ten years out of date.'

'I'm afraid I must circulate and can't discuss these with you.'

Not long after this it was reported that frank discussions had taken place with the Presidents of the Medical Royal Colleges!

There was a strong move, mainly by Margaret Turner-Warwick and Peter Lachmann, the President of the Royal College of Pathologists, to form an Academy of Medicine in place of the Conference. I was opposed to this as I thought that an Academy of Medicine may not have its membership solely vested in the Presidents and such an Academy could become the negotiating body with the Department of Health. This would demote the voice and the power of individual colleges. I stated my opposition. No such body has yet been formed but the Conference has been renamed the Academy of Medical Royal Colleges. This is acceptable.

I am a poor politician. I don't think naturally in terms of politics and a major failing is my tendency to speak my mind frankly. This is often an instinctive decision and not necessarily thought through in terms of politics. This is not a virtue and I regret it may have lost me support at times and possibly friendships. A good example of this concerned Sir Robert Kilpatrick, President of the General Medical Council at the time. He came to the Conference to discuss his Performance Review Procedure, about which he was very enthusiastic. This was concerned with tightening up our dealing with poor performance by doctors. There is no doubt the profession has been lax in dealing with colleagues whose performance is, for one reason or another, less than satisfactory. If this is due to illness the mechanism is moderately good, but for reasons of professional competence or unacceptable behaviour remedial action is too long delayed or even not taken. The Performance Review Procedure requires action to be taken directly to the General Medical Council who will deal with the matter. This seems to be reasonable and indeed a worthy fashion in which to deal with a difficult problem. However I had anxieties. I asked questions.

'Sir Robert, what types of performance can be reported as unsatisfactory?'

'Incompetence, rudeness, unsatisfactory behaviour in general.'

'What about mistakes?'

'No, it must be consistent incompetence.'

That seems very reasonable.

'What action can be taken?'

'The doctor in question may need treatment, may need retraining or may be removed from the register.'

'Who can report the doctor to the General Medical Council?'

'Many people – patients, nurses, colleagues.'

'What about lay managers?'

'Yes, they can report unacceptable behaviour.'

I had anxieties that although the theory was good and acceptable, personal vendettas, common in medicine at a hospital level, could cause problems. Jealous doctors could be a problem. I was worried also that managers might wish to silence or rid themselves of a difficult doctor.

I was unsure of how it would work. I wished that such issues could be dealt with at a local level by a strong medical committee, but I have to admit that such was not the case in the past. However I made my views known. At the moment I'm unaware how the Performance Review Procedure is working, but I do know I was the only questioning voice at the meeting. I also know I displeased Sir Robert and may have lost his friendship.

Terence English was President of the Royal College of Surgeons for the same three years of my Presidency 1989–1992. Terence came from South Africa and in 1954 obtained a BSc from Witwatersrand University. He qualified in medicine in 1962 from Guy's Hospital Medical School. I first met Terence in 1966 when he was surgical registrar at the Bolingbroke Hospital where I had three consultant sessions. I was leaving the hospital at about 8.00 p.m. having just given a tutorial to candidates for the Membership of the Royal College of Physicians, and I met Terence on the stairs going to the X-ray Department.

'Are you going to the X-ray Department?' I asked.

'Yes, I've admitted a young child with acute abdominal pain and vomiting.'

'What did you find on examination?'

'That's the strange thing. She has a temperature and I suspect an inflammation but there is no abdominal tenderness and although an appendicitis seems likely she hasn't got the abdominal signs of it.'

'Make sure you get an abdominal X-ray in both the erect and supine positions. Would you like me to see the films with you?'

'Thank you, please.'

The films were extraordinary. There was a small loop of bowel with a fluid level lying high on the right side of the abdomen. This could easily have been overlooked but with the symptoms the child had, the presence of fever yet no abdominal signs, I suspected an unusual appendicitis. For reasons too complicated for this text I diagnosed a high retrocaecal abscess (lying toward the back), due to a ruptured appendix. I told Terence my diagnosis and wondered whether or not he believed me, but indeed that is what he found at operation. I've always thought this was one of my most clever diagnoses. I've used these films in teaching the interpretation of acute abdominal disorders for years.

Terence became a consultant in cardiothoracic surgery in Papworth Hospital in Cambridge. He was also Director of Papworth Heart Transplant Unit and his reputation was international. He was awarded many Fellowships and in 1984–1985 was President of the International Society of Heart Transplantation. He was knighted in 1991.

He is a charming, handsome man with a keen sense of humour and a warm personality. He captained Guy's Hospital Rugby Football team in 1959. St Mary's didn't win the Hospitals Rugby Cup that year. Until 1997, Guy's have won the cup thirty one times and St Mary's thirty two. St Thomas's are third having won it fifteen times. I wish Terence had been a student at St Mary's!

Margaret Turner-Warwick, whose mother before marriage was Maud Baden-Powell, coincided with both Terence and me in being President of the Royal College of Physicians from 1989–1992. She is an extraordinary woman, warm hearted, good natured and congenial. She is superintelligent, efficient and effective. She was Professor of Medicine at the Brompton Hospital and Dean of the Cardiothoracic Institute from 1984–1987. She was President of the British Thoracic Society from 1982–1985. As well as her numerous Fellowships she is an Honorary Bencher of the Middle Temple. Margaret has written extensively on chest disease and she too has a well acknowledged international reputation. She was made a Dame of the British Empire (DBE) in 1991.

Margaret is strongly anti-smoking, and on one occasion after dinner in the Royal College of Surgeons, Terence English, Stanley Simmons and I each had a cigar. The Royal College of Surgeons at the time did not have a no smoking policy, mainly because of Lord Porritt, who was a committed cigarette smoker. This has since changed. Margaret looked at us and said,

'Well I suppose a cigar after dinner might be acceptable.'

It was an act of kindness for her to say so, feeling as she does, and it eased any tension there could have been. Strangely it was one of the last cigars I ever smoked. Margaret is married to Richard Turner-Warwick, emeritus senior surgeon and urologist to the Middlesex Hospital. Richard was on the council of the Royal College of Surgeons and was President of the British Association of Urological Surgeons. He too has numerous Fellowships and a worldwide reputation. While at Oxford he was a member of the University Boat Race crew.

Each Christmas in retirement I receive a card from Margaret and Richard on which is reproduced one of Margaret's water colour paintings which are all of a high quality.

Chapter 6

Presidential Activities

Most medical colleges are criticized. It's impossible to please everyone. The English medical colleges are situated in London and the most common criticism is that each is a London based club. This criticism comes mainly from non-London based Fellows. The Royal College of Radiologists is the only radiological college in the United Kingdom, but the Royal College of Physicians has a college in Edinburgh as does the Royal College of Surgeons.

I have looked at the source of the Presidents of the Royal College of Radiologists since 1975, and of the eleven, only four were based in London. There were twelve Wardens of whom only four were based in London. There were eight Vice-Presidents of Clinical Radiology and only two were based in London and of eight Vice-presidents in Clinical Oncology, only two were based in London. So most of the senior officers of the College were practising medicine outside London. This trend is also reflected in the membership of the college committees. Nonetheless when I took over as President I was aware that many Fellows in the counties of England, in Northern Ireland, Scotland and Wales felt remote from the College and thought they had no input into college policies. I decided early on to visit each region of the United Kingdom to meet with Fellows and have a question and answer session. I wished to bring the College out to them. I always brought another college officer with me. It meant a great deal of traveling and time, but I think the time used was worthwhile. I think the meetings were successful, but I remember one Scot in Edinburgh interrupting me in mid sentence, saying, 'We are no' concerned what goes on the other side of that border.' Nobody in the large audience of Scottish Fellows contradicted him and somehow I felt he might have spoken for them. I expected trouble in Glasgow but the reception was excellent, and they rolled out the red carpet for us. Perhaps they wished to be different from Edinburgh!

I had four Vice-Presidents during my term as President. Ian Kerr was the first. He and I had been friends for years. We both belonged to the

Shadows Radiological Travelling Club and together with our wives had many happy hours together. Ian did his pre-clinical studies in Cambridge and his clinical studies in Guy's Hospital Medical School in London. He obtained his Membership of the Royal College of Physicians in 1956 and his Fellowship in Radiology in 1962.

When we were beginning our specialization in radiology the first trainee posts we applied for were at Guy's Hospital. It was then I first met Ian. Eight candidates were short listed, all with higher qualifications, seven being Members of the Royal College of Physicians and me being a Fellow of the Royal College of Surgeons. On the day of the selection committee, seven of us were sitting together in the main office in Guy's waiting to be called in for interview, when the eighth appeared. When he entered the office, the secretaries all smiled, rose and came over to him, shaking his hand, laughing and chatting. I turned to the candidate next to me.

'Do you know who is going to get this job?'

'Of course not. How could I?'

'I'll tell you.'

'Who?'

'The man that just came in.'

It was Ian Kerr who was well known and liked in Guy's. Rightly he got the post, Ian was well qualified and indeed a Guy's man. It was reasonable for him to get the post, but I worried that a Bart's man would get the Bart's job, a Middlesex man the Middlesex job and a Thomas's man the St Thomas's job. I had come from a Dublin medical school. Thank God for St Mary's because even though a St Mary's man was a candidate I got the trainee job and as they say, 'the rest is history'.

Ian has had a very successful career. He became a specialist in chest disease and a consultant at the Brompton Hospital in London. He also had sessions at King Edward VII Hospital in Midhurst and sessions in private practice. He published papers on chest disease in reputable medical journals and was invited to join the Fleishner Society, a prestigious international society of chest radiologists. Ian was editor of *Clinical Radiology*, the scientific journal of the Royal College of Radiologists from 1983 to 1987, and Vice-President of the College from 1987 to 1989.

Ian has a quiet contemplative personality, quite unlike me, and together the balance was good. When he retired he went to live in

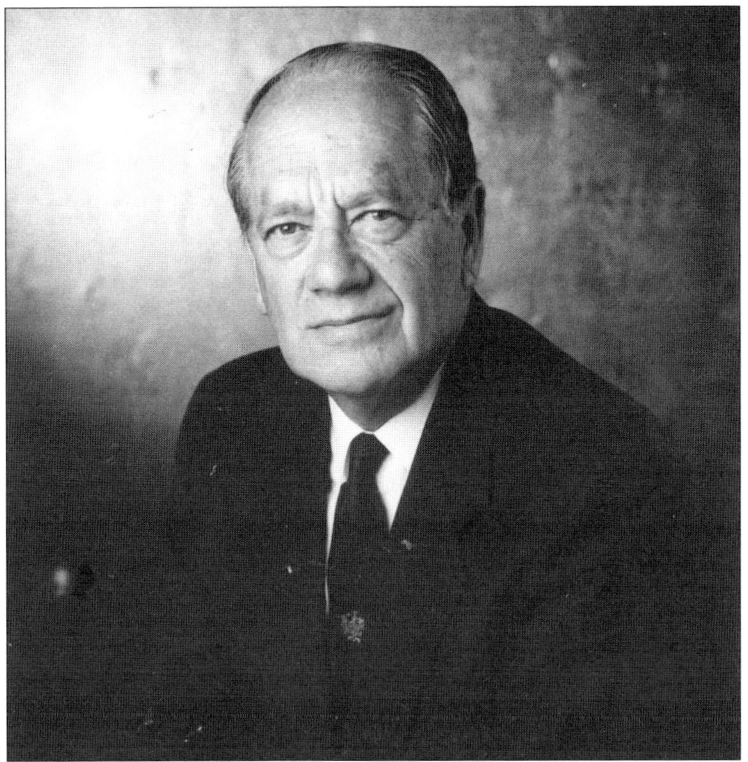

Dr Ian Kerr. Consultant Radiologist Brompton Hospital, London. Past Vice-President Royal College of Radiologists

Scotland near Inverness, the home of his ancestors, where he is happy, especially when playing golf. Nesta his wife, also medically qualified, came to most of the college meetings and the college dinners. I remember well my first conversation with her when we were juniors in the late 1950s.

'What children have you got, Nesta?'

'Two boys.'

'I've only got daughters, four of them. It seems I can only make girls.'

'I would like to have a daughter.'

'Nesta, we should get together. I could give you a daughter.'

'Why not, Oscar!'

We have laughed about this for forty years. Nesta often says when we meet, 'I'm still waiting'.

The second Vice-President I had was Thelma Bates, a clinical oncologist. Thelma was consultant in Radiotherapy to St Thomas's

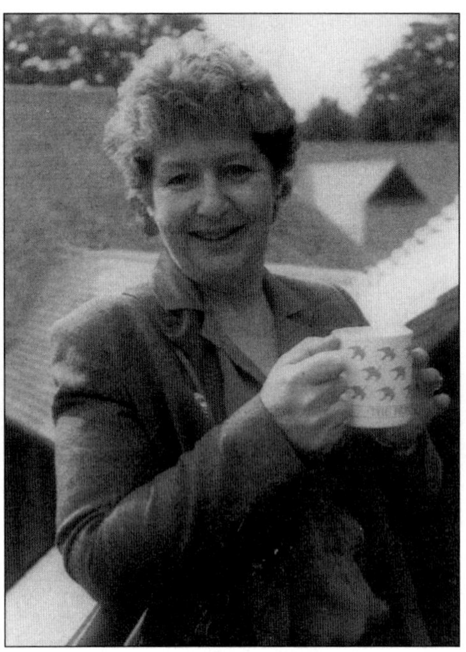

Dr Thelma Bates. Consultant in Clinical Oncology, St Thomas's Hospital. Past Vice-President Royal College of Radiologists

Hospital, London. She is a kind, caring woman, full of energy and humour. She is highly intelligent and skilled in her specialty, and with an interest in the theatre has a number of well known actors as patients. She became Chairman of the Health Committee of the General Medical Council (GMC), and a member of the Criminal Injuries Compensation Appeals Committee. During my Presidency she was a great support to me. There was one incident in particular. At a time when anxiety was being expressed by the public and the media about the dangers of irradiation, diagnostic radiology especially came under scrutiny and patients voiced anxiety about radiological investigations. I was invited to speak on the Jimmy Young radio show. This was an opportunity to put people's minds at rest. I've given many lectures, after dinner speeches and have been televised but never experienced a live question and answer session on radio,where I had to think on my feet and formulate a sensible and accurate answer in seconds. This request made me nervous.

'Thelma, I'm frightened.'

'Whatever for?'

'I don't know the questions he'll ask, and must answer quickly and correctly without adding to people's alarm.'

'You'll have no problem.'

'There may be millions of people listening and I mustn't let the college down, and must reassure patients and potential patients.'

'You're the very man to do it well.'

'I'm still frightened.'

'Oscar, I'll come with you and you'll be great.'

Thelma came with me to the BBC, encouraging me all the time. Her support was enormous and I emotionally relied on her. She sat in the adjoining room watching and listening to my performance. Jimmy Young was charming and all went well. I've been grateful to Thelma for this ever since. For me she was the right person at the right time.

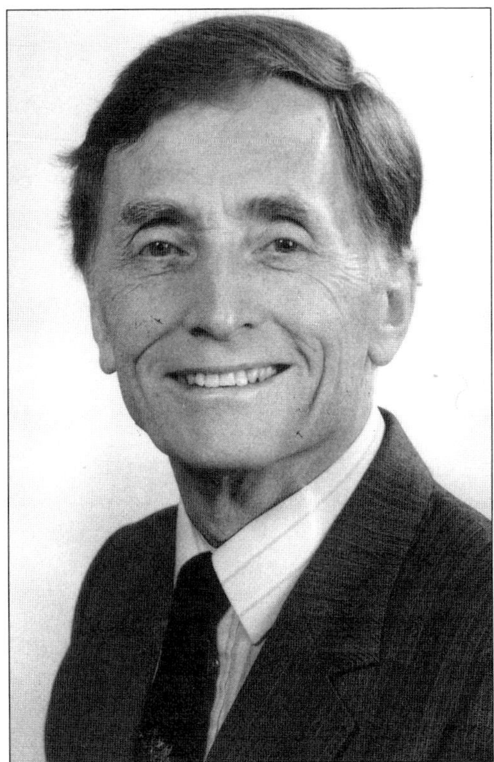

Dr Dennis Stoker. Consultant Radiologist Royal National Orthopaedic Hospital. Past Vice-President Royal College of Radiologists

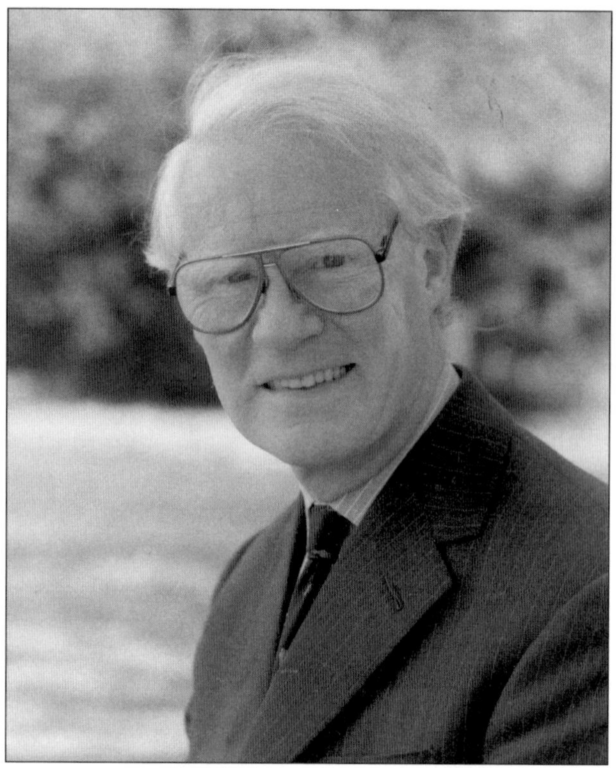

Sir Christopher Paine. Consultant in Clinical Oncology. Past President Royal College of Radiologists

The next Vice-President was Dennis Stoker. Dennis is an extraordinary man who had an extraordinary career. He qualified in medicine in 1951 from Guy's Hospital Medical School, and obtained his Membership of the Royal College of Physicians in 1958. He spent his early career as a consultant physician in the medical branch of the Royal Air Force from 1951 to 1968. When he retired from the RAF, still a relatively young man at forty, he decided to specialize in radiology. He began his studies for the Fellowship in Radiology which he got in 1971. Dennis took to his new specialty with enormous enthusiasm and skill and soon was a consultant in the Royal National Orthopaedic Hospital and later Dean of the Institute of Orthopaedics in the University of London. He was made a Fellow of the Royal College of Surgeons ad eundem in 1992. Having had two careers, in his second he became the most distinguished expert of his time in the radiology of bone and joint disease. His reputation in this field was acknowledged internationally. He wrote and lectured extensively. Dennis too, as Vice-President in 1990 to 1991 was a great choice to balance me. He is quiet by nature, is a clear thinker, has a placid temperament and an earnest manner.

For the year 1991 to 1992, Chris Paine was the Vice-President. Chris qualified in Oxford in 1961 and obtained his Membership of the Royal College of Physicians in 1964. He specialized in Radiotherapy and took his Fellowship in 1969, in which he obtained the Rohan Williams Medal. During his career he was District General Manager in the Oxford Health Authority and Director of Clinical Studies in Oxford University. He followed me as President of the Royal College of Radiologists in 1992. Later he was President of the Royal Society of Medicine.

Chris is a rare medical man, having an instinct for issues of political significance and an administrative ability. His assessment of difficult issues is never clouded by emotion but led by a clear incisive mind of great value whether as a member of a committee or its chairman. He was chosen to chair the committee that rationalized the oncology treatment centres in London and was awarded the KBE in 1995. It was Chris who accompanied me on my regional visit to Scotland when we visited Edinburgh, Glasgow and Aberdeen. We arrived in Aberdeen in a fog which grounded all planes, but we managed to get back to London by train.

Chris and his wife live near Minehead in Somerset and we only meet occasionally now at College affairs.

For a long time I thought the juniors in the specialty should have a direct voice in the college. Calling them juniors seems so ridiculous as they invariably were doubly qualified in medicine and held registrar and senior registrar posts. The junior title merely meant they had not yet reached consultant status, but they were men and women of experience. I spoke to Council about forming a Junior Radiologists Forum, and had no difficulty in getting agreement. Each region of England, Northern Ireland, Scotland and Wales would have a representative in clinical radiology and clinical oncology from whom an Executive Forum would be picked. The chairman would sit on Council and bring to Council the views and opinions of the juniors from throughout the United Kingdom. This has been very successful and thank God, was one of my good ideas!

I thought another good idea was to form a Friends of the Royal College of Radiologists Association. My plan was to get wives of consultants and other well wishers to support the College throughout the United Kingdom, to organize fundraising events, whist drives, golf tournaments, coffee mornings, dances and the like and in raising funds for research also advertise the College and the specialty of radiology. Most of the population don't understand the work of a radiologist and what part he plays in medicine. Most of the population don't know the difference between a radiologist and a radiographer or what the relationship is between them. Most of the population don't know the part played by radiologists in the treatment of cancer, heart and vascular disease, the great killers.

I thought the most suitable person to chair such an association was Rose Roebuck. Rose is the wife of Eric Roebuck, a consultant radiologist in Nottingham who plays a major role in the fight against cancer as an expert in breast screening. Eric writes many scientific papers on breast screening and organizes superb training courses, which are among the most popular courses in the United Kingdom. Eric was Registrar of the College from 1985 to 1990. I remember well my conversation with Rose.

'I want to form a Friends of the Royal College of Radiologists Association, would you be interested in chairing it?'

'Tell me more.'

'I want the Friends to raise funds for the college, but also to raise the profile of the College throughout the United Kingdom.'

'I would be interested in doing that.'

'You would have your own agenda. Do what you wish. We will not interfere with you, but may I suggest you get a representative from each region, but I can assure you the entire running of it will be up to you.'

'What about the finance?'

'Once you get running you should be self supporting and any money you raise must go to the College and the decision for its use will be up to Council.'

'Oscar, I'll do it.'

The Friends got going while I was President and it was very successful. Fund-raising stalls were manned by volunteers at each major College meeting and indeed at meetings of the British Institute of Radiology, and were supported by all participants. The stall even helped

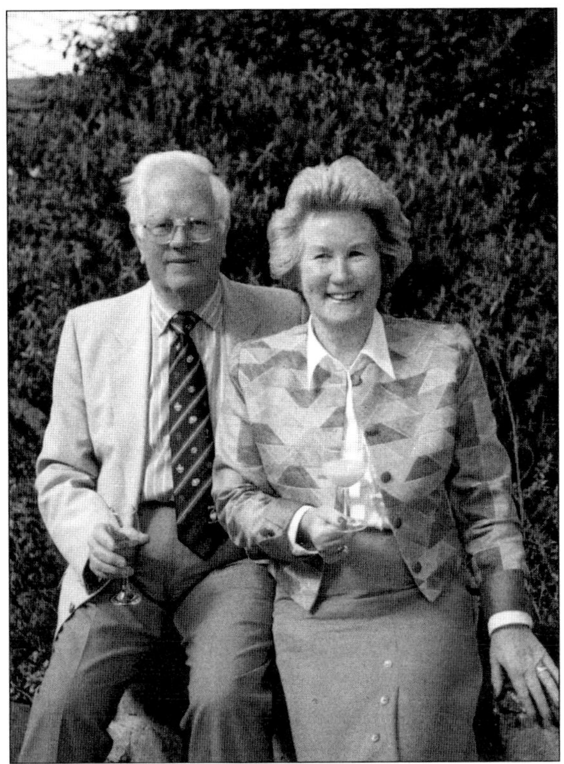

Dr Eric Roebuck. Consultant Radiologist. Past Registrar Royal College of Radiologists and Rose Roebuck, Chair of The Friends of the Royal College of Radiologists

the image of the College with our own Fellows. Funds were raised by Rose organizing a large number of events in the United Kingdom which included golf tournaments. She did a magnificent job.

At some stage, I can't remember the exact time, an X Appeal committee was formed which took over the major fund raising for research. This was principally under the chairmanship of Norman Howard, a clinical oncologist. I heard some days ago that he is retiring from the post and Terence Priestman, another oncologist, is taking his place.

However the X Appeal continues and many thousands of pounds have been raised to support research. The Fellows of the College have to submit their research projects for examination to qualify for funding. Having lost the Friends I was dismayed but take some pride in that the X Appeal continues.

I had another anxiety that the College had no line of communication with the radiologists in the armed forces, yet they were Fellows of the

College. I thought it might be helpful to them and cement our relationship if a representative could sit on Council as an observer. I wrote to the Director General of Medical Services for the Armed Forces, and in due time a representative was named and attended. A scientific meeting with the military radiologists also was arranged and went well. I believe that since my Presidency this representation has lapsed. It seems some of my ideas remained but others perished.

A successful venture was to take a team of lecturers to India. This was funded by the British Council. We lectured to hundreds of radiologists in different centres for sixteen days. We visited Bombay, Hyderabad, Calcutta, Delhi, Jaipur and Agra. In Calcutta we attended the Annual Congress of the Indian Radiological and Imaging Association. The President of this Association was Major General Dhawan, a radiologist who had been the senior physician in the Indian Armed Forces. He is an intelligent, charming and courteous gentleman. His quiet speaking manner hides the strong leadership in his character. In our lectures and tutorials we covered most of the specialities within radiology, including ultrasound and computed tomography (CT scanning). The Indian doctors were touchingly enthusiastic, remarkably keen and attentive. They asked questions continually, even during breaks for refreshments, lunch or dinner. They crowded around us constantly. Such was their thirst for teaching.

There were official lunches and dinners daily and our diet was one curry after another. Each curry no matter how different had one thing in common. They were the hottest I've ever tasted. As a result I had indigestion and diarrhoea for sixteen days. I spoke to one of my colleagues who had experience climbing in the Himalaya.

'Philip, I can't walk.'

'I know what you've got.'

'What?'

'A ring burn!'

A ring burn described it perfectly. It was painful even to wipe my bottom. I also had pain in my lower chest from reflux which burnt the lower end of my oesophagus (gullet). At one dinner toward the end of our stay I developed acute chest pain. The Indian doctors gathered around in great concern.

'Oh, Dr Craig, you've had a heart attack. You've got acute angina or a coronary thrombosis.'

'I haven't. I have reflux oesophagitis from the hot curries.'

They didn't understand how their curry could possibly do that.

'You'd better be careful. It is surely a heart attack.'

'Well whatever, I'm going to bed.'

I went to bed but they came to my room at intervals asking me more radiological questions. If I'd had a heart attack their insistence would have killed me. Even my colleagues who liked hot curries got tired of them and at one official dinner hid their full plates under the table. I was anxious lest our hosts noticed this or even by accident stood on the plates, but nothing disastrous happened. At another dinner we were amused when Major General Dhawan before giving his official speech rose and said, 'Will the servants please withdraw.'

We all smiled at each other and wondered what reception this would have if we said the same thing in the United Kingdom.

I was so impressed by the Major General, his reception for us all and his anglophile feelings as well as his intellect, that I invited him to come as our official guest to the next Annual Meeting of the Royal College of Radiologists and to be the guest speaker at the Annual Dinner. He came with his wife, a gynaecologist with a forceful character, to stay in our home in Cheam. While they were with us, before the Annual Dinner, there was a meeting of the Twenty Five Club, in Cambridge. We brought them as our guests to the meeting held in the Garden House Hotel. I think the General enjoyed the scientific meeting and the social occasion and Nancy entertained his wife. The members of the Twenty Five Club made them both very welcome. The Annual Dinner of the College was held in Edinburgh that year and we brought the General and his wife with us by train. One of the great surprises I got was to discover that the General hadn't been to the United Kingdom before and so his trip was all the more enjoyable. He spoke well at the dinner about Anglo-Indian relationships in medicine. Kenneth Calman the Chief Medical Officer was the other guest and his speech was excellent and humorous. I thought I gave one of my poorest speeches that night and it certainly was too long.

In India I had to give an enormous number of speeches, sometimes without any prior notice. On one occasion the official speaker didn't turn up and just before we sat down to dinner I was asked to speak instead. I have no skill in impromptu speeches. I like to prepare my speeches well in advance. I warned my colleagues that at some time, someone would question why we taught on so modern a subject and such sophisticated technology when what they needed in India was basic medicine and clean water. I was right because while in Calcutta, the Minister of Health said,

'Thank you for coming to India. Thank you for your expertise and your teaching. You bring us the latest in technological medicine but I must point out that our needs before that are immunization programmes, modern sanitation, hygiene and clean water.'

I replied, 'Yes you are right, but Indian radiologists wish to learn the latest techniques and are enthusiastic about progressing in their specialty. That is their duty and what they will do best. They are not the ones to dig wells and others will bring immunization programmes and skills in preventative medicine.'

I had to say that, but what I saw in India made radiological techniques a luxury. The streets were lined by make shift shelters of sacking, below which lived families, who scavenged food from rubbish tips. They ate what they could and defecated where they were. At night bodies lay on the pavements head to toe covered by sacks, some just sleeping, some dead. We didn't know which until morning. Flies were everywhere, blindness was everywhere. Those not physically blind were emotionally blind. There was an atmosphere of hopelessness. Leprous arms banged on car windows begging for help of any kind. Children in rags roamed the streets. Tuberculous patients lay on the steps of hospitals unable to get in. The extravagance of the hotels close by seemed indecent and the wealth of many was such a contrast as to be unbearable. No blame can be laid at anyone's door, as the task to care for the millions of people is so enormous. It seems impossible to solve. It is tragedy on a grand scale.

However there was also beauty. The beauty was seen in the dignity of the women in the fields, even the most lowly, walking straight in colourful saris, with beautiful dark sad eyes, in young children unaware of the life ahead – smiling, in growing girls and boys uniformed for school, anticipating a better life for them and India. There was beauty in the hills, in the fields and buildings, in palaces and fortresses and in the Taj Mahal. There was beauty in the glimpses of the past. India is full of contrasts, of luxury and lack.

We travelled throughout the countryside in a small bus. Helen Carty, a paediatric radiologist from Liverpool was the only volunteer to sit in the front beside the driver. His maniacal driving scattered everything and everybody in his path while his hand pumped the horn in harmony with his shouting, while we all sat bolt upright in fear. Internal air flights caused Nancy and me similar fear.

When we left India we were each given what they said was a special present. It was an ornate gold coloured clock. We carried these carefully to the airport. At the airport the shops were full of them!

The following year we had another invitation to lecture in India. The tour was repeated but fearful of more ring burns and reflux oesophagitis I let a colleague go in my place. I'm glad we did these lecture tours. They were highly successful and we taught and encouraged more radiologists than could possibly have come to the United Kingdom for instruction.

I'm not surprised that another of my ideas wasn't fulfilled and likely won't ever be fulfilled. For many years I've wished radiology in the United Kingdom to be represented by one major body formed by the amalgamation of the Royal College of Radiologists and the British Institute of Radiology. There are major problems to such a union, but I wished a dialogue to commence. A major problem is that the Royal College of Radiologists is confined to Members and Fellows who are medically qualified. The British Institute of Radiology (BIR) is the oldest radiological society in the United Kingdom and is open to radiologists, radiographers, physicists, nuclear medicine specialists and those involved in commerce associated with radiology. The BIR does a sterling job arranging lectures, seminars, and large scientific meetings but has no examining body and cannot issue degrees or diplomas. The BIR has no political voice with government or with the other medical colleges. The Royal College of Radiologists also arranges lectures, tutorials, seminars and scientific meetings and has a political voice. It is also an examining body which provides a Fellowship which is a recommendation for every consultant post in clinical radiology and clinical oncology. The BIR building is next door to the college and only a wall separates them. I wished to see the wall removed. I mentioned this possibility at every opportunity in after dinner speeches but found little support. There was no support from the BIR who believed the College would dominate. I could see a large College with many faculties housed in an imposing building, financially and politically stronger than the separate bodies. Perhaps the concept is flawed and the status quo will remain.

Chapter 7

Medical Litigation

DURING MY MEDICAL CAREER I was invited to sit on the Cases Committee of the Medical Protection Society, Hallam Street, London. This Society dealt with medical litigation and advised and defended doctors in court. I sat on the Council of the Society and chaired the Cases Committee for many years. Some years ago I travelled from London to give medical evidence in the Dublin law courts near to the Halfpenny Bridge. When the solicitor, a young lady, was driving me back to the airport, we passed the Halipenny Bridge over the River Liffey. I asked her to slow down for me to have a good look at it.

'This bridge is very important to me.'

'Why's that?'

'My wife and I became engaged on this bridge while we were medical students. I gave her my signet ring and asked her to wear it on the appropriate finger until I could get the money for the proper ring for her. That was in 1948, fifty four years ago.'

' That's very romantic.'

'I've always wanted a print of this bridge, but could never find one.'

A few months later a parcel arrived at my home in Cheam. Inside was a letter from the solicitor,

> Dear Dr Craig,
>
> I remember you had an affection for the Halfpenny Bridge. I couldn't find a print, but enclosed is a watercolour of it which I think is more beautiful than a print, and I want you to have it.

I was astonished and touched by this act of kindness. It hangs in our breakfast room and I look at it each day.

I've enjoyed my work in the field of medical litigation, although giving expert evidence in court can be daunting. Barristers have intelligent, sharp minds, are skilled in cross examination and sensitive to any weakness in an expert witness. They can ruthlessly expose any flaw in one's argument. It is of course a confrontational system. Barristers who undertake a medical case are invariably well read in the subject of that particular case. The judge must base his verdict on the arguments presented by the prosecution and defence, which in turn can rest on the quality of the evidence given by the medical experts.

It's a sad fact that litigation against the medical profession has increased considerably in the last few decades, following the pattern in the United States of America. I am driven to the conclusion that today most doctors can expect to have at least one allegation for negligence against him or her in their medical lifetime. Medicine is not an exact science and the human body doesn't respond to medicine or treatments in a set pattern. However nor is the doctor free from error. Many mishaps are unavoidable and can be complications of drugs or treatments. It is often the case that the plaintiff cannot distinguish between an acceptable complication or what is due to an avoidable error. Neither is the law free from error and I've known unjust and indeed incorrect judgements in court. It's possible for the judge to be influenced by the convincing acting of an expert witness even though the opinion given is far outside that accepted by the medical profession. We must live with this in our present system in the same way a batsman in cricket must abide by the decision of the umpire. I find it easy to accept the latter, but medical litigation is not a sport.

I think it must be true that most if not all doctors are lucky to avoid an accusation of negligence at some stage in their lives. I can remember some personal cases where litigation could have occurred even though I was acting at all times in good faith and with due care. I have recalled elsewhere one in general practice. There were two possible cases when I was a surgeon in the Royal Air Force Hospital in Ely, Cambridgeshire. The hospital, apart from air force personnel, also took civilians referred from local general practitioners. The nearest civilian hospital was in Cambridge about eighteen miles away. The arrangement to take civilian patients helped the general practitioners but also the RAF specialists. They gained experience particularly in patients of the age group not available in the forces. However both the cases I quote here were young.

An eighteen-year-old man was admitted from a local practitioner complaining of acute abdominal pain, vomiting and fever. These are the features of many acute abdominal emergencies whatever the cause. He lay still in bed and couldn't move without agony. On examination his abdomen was tender and rigid all over. There were no localizing points to suggest an origin for the trouble. The diagnosis of generalized peritonitis was easy but what was the cause? To establish the cause before operating was in many ways crucial. The history was vague with no past indigestion or vomiting and the present situation had occured suddenly and out of the blue as it were. There were no clues. I decided that the most common cause of an acute abdominal emergency in a male patient of this age was a ruptured appendix. I took him to theatre and made an incision over the appendix. I was surprised and dismayed to find he had a normal appendix. What should I do now? With a surgical retractor I lifted up the edges of the surgical incision to get a better look and saw some flaky white debris in the upper abdomen. My God, he had a perforated duodenal ulcer. I couldn't reach it from this incision. What now? I closed the appendix incision and made a long upper abdominal incision, technically called a right upper paramedian incision that would allow better access. I located the perforated duodenal ulcer and successfully closed the perforation. He woke up to find two incisions for the one operation. The major error I made was making the assumption he had a perforated appendix and compounded that by making an initial small incision over the appendix. This was due to my inexperience but really shouldn't have happened. In the first instance I should have made a vertical paramedian incision to allow for an adequate assessment of the abdomen. He did very well and was discharged fit and had no complications. However despite doing well and being 'saved' from his acute emergency, in today's litigious climate he might have sued me.

One Wednesday afternoon, sports day in the RAF, a young man of seventeen was admitted with a history of passing blood in his urine. He had been playing football and was the goalkeeper of his team. While saving a ball on the ground he had been kicked in the right flank. Just after the game he passed blood in the toilet. An ambulance was called and he was brought to the hospital in Ely where I was on surgical duty. There was little doubt he had received a severe injury to his left kidney, but how severe could not be told at this stage. I admitted him and took all the necessary precautions with regular and repeated blood pressure readings, pulse monitoring and the collection of all his urine for examination. I immediately contacted the department of radiology and requested an X-ray examination of his kidneys. At that time in 1954 there was no ultrasound available. The department of radiology gave me an appointment for the examination which was some days later.

However the bleeding stopped and the blood pressure and pulse were normal. He had no abdominal pain and no other physical signs of note. Two days later I was going on leave. I passed him over to the surgeon on duty for me.

On my return I asked how the boy was.

'We had a terrible time. On Saturday evening he had a torrential haemorrhage, passing pure blood, and his blood pressure fell dramatically. I had to rush him to the theatre.'

'My God, is he alright?

'Yes, he's recovering in the ward, but it's been difficult.'

'What did you find?'

'I did an anterior approach to his kidney, also to get a good look in his abdomen in case of trauma to other organs. I found his right kidney lacerated in several areas and sufficiently damaged to require removal. Before doing so I felt for his left kidney to see that it was normal as I had no knowledge of it in the absence of a radiological examination. My God, I couldn't find a left kidney. I thought of the possibility of a pelvic kidney, rare though they are, and felt carefully in his pelvis.

There was none there. The awful fact I faced was that he had only one kidney and it was severely damaged. I spent a great deal of time repairing the lacerations as best I could. By the grace of God, he's doing well but we've had the additional problem of keeping his electrolyte balance stable.'

Absence of a kidney is rare but well known. Today we would have had an immediate ultrasound examination which would have demonstrated the degree of damage to the kidney and in addition would have revealed to us the absence of the right kidney and the presence or otherwise of a pelvic kidney. It's remarkable how wonderful these investigations are and what a great advance they have made in patient care. This information would be available within minutes. In addition an isotope investigation would have demonstrated the function in the damaged kidney, another valuable asset.

What was my mistake, if there was one? The only investigation available at the time was the radiological examination by means of an intravenous injection and the X-ray visualization of the kidneys. This would have shown the damage to the right kidney and the absence of the left kidney. It would also have shown the function remaining in the right kidney. I should have insisted on having the X-ray examination done immediately and have spoken to the radiological consultant to inform him of the urgency of the case. I failed to do this. Would it have made any difference to the outcome? Perhaps not, but it would have helped to have been forewarned and not to have faced the situation for the first time at the operation. It was fortunate that the surgeon who took over from me was experienced and made all the right decisions.

The patient made a full recovery and was discharged fit.

Medicine has its funny as well as its serious side.

When taking a surgical clinic in Ely the nurse brought in a middle-aged man to see me. Having greeted him I enquired,

'What's the trouble?'

'Doctor, I've got noodles.'

'Noodles!'

'Yes, Doctor, noodles.'

This really foxed me and I looked at him for some time totally confused but expecting him to enlarge on this. He just stared back and said nothing. I decided to try again.

'What sort of noodles?'

'Big ones.'

'Where?'

'On my feet.'

I thought I'd better look.

'Show them to me.'

I saw the lumps and suddenly all seemed clear.

'You mean nodules.'

'That right Doctor – noodles.'

He smiled, happy at last I understood what noodles were.

A case where I did well but was thwarted was an eighty-year-old woman referred with abdominal pain, vomiting and fever. In this case however she had a large tender lump in the lower right hand side of her abdomen. This pain had been present for days and she was very ill. She certainly needed an immediate operation. I took her to theatre and on opening the abdomen found the largest appendix I'd ever seen.

It was red, inflamed and seemed on the point of bursting. It was an infected mucocoele of the appendix filled with pus.

I said to my assistant, 'This is a lovely case for our next clinical meeting. We must keep the specimen.'

I clamped the base of the appendix and removed it carefully. It was a prize specimen. I put the removed appendix with the clamp still in place in a receiving bowl and handed it to the nurse to take to the sluice room. I closed the abdomen carefully, very satisfied I'd done a good job. I went to the sluice room to view my prize. Horror of horrors, I found a shrivelled deflated appendix. The nurse had removed the clamp on its base and the pus contents had all drained away destroying my specimen. I tried to present it at the clinical meeting but telling the story was feeble and sounded like the angler telling the story of his great catch, but the fish got away. The patient did very well with no complications and went home happy.

Experience in medicine is invaluable and we learn something from each patient. Later in my career when I was a consultant radiologist at St Mary's Hospital, Paddington, I had a most unusual patient who taught me much about personal courage. She was a private patient I saw in the Lindo Wing of the hospital. She was thin, so very thin. There was nothing about her body to steal attention from her face. Her smile was friendly, natural and warm. It seemed to spread into the surroundings and suck you in. Her eyes were large, dark, vibrant and exciting. Her cheekbones were high and prominent, above a wide mouth, full with large soft lips. This was rare beauty crowned by jet black hair, shining, straight and short. Her light coffee coloured skin looked fragile and had a lustre that tempted touch. When she spoke her eyes held fast to mine and danced with fun and merriment.

Of course I recognized her at once having seen her so often in the fashion magazines, and sometimes on the cover in a dramatic pose. She was one of the first coloured models with this level of success in the United Kingdom. How well I remember how compelling those magazine covers were. But I'll never forget her as a patient.

When she spoke I was disturbed immediately. It wasn't just the high toned singing voice, but the bad grammar and foul language she used. I couldn't join this voice and language to her beauty or to the warmth that this young woman spread about her, enveloping me. In time I got used to it, and then barely noticed it, so strong was her appeal.

As we talked I learnt about the poverty of her Jamaican family. I asked myself, as I've done many times since, how did she manage to become such a success in so hard a world. The clothes she was wearing now, off duty as it were, were ordinary, a thigh length jumper, over designer jeans. They were so unlike the clothes she modelled but didn't detract from her allure. She moved like a lean lithe animal, and I smiled as I thought of the cat walk.

Her male companions were flashy. I disliked them immediately. I decided they were parasites living on her substantial earnings. I never changed my mind about them. Their slick smoothness and aftershave sweetness offends me still, years later.

In the consulting room I questioned her fully.

'Doctor, it's the diarrhoea.'

She wasn't one to beat about the bush and came quickly to the point, using her colourful language.

'I know every bog in the big cities all over Europe. I pose in a square in Venice and after each photograph, rush to the bog. I do the same in Paris, Rome, Berlin, Florence and Vienna.'

She paused for a moment.

'It wasn't so bad when I was fourteen.'

I had to hide my anxiety, as I'd done for so many others. With her I found it difficult. She had this problem for years and it had to be one of the chronic large bowel inflammations. The examination I had to do would confirm this and show me the extent to which it had spread. She must have known the seriousness of her problem for a long time, but I didn't insult her by asking why she had waited.

Perhaps I knew the answer. The examination confirmed the diagnosis, and showed extensive bowel involvement.

She responded to treatment and passed out of my life. Some years later she returned looking no different. Her smile and physical appearance were as captivating. Again she had male companions, different faces, but the same expensive clothes, crocodile shoes, sweet sick smell and Rolex watches. I found I hadn't lost my prejudices.

'I'm having trouble again, but this time I've pain.'

I hoped my face didn't betray my sinking heart as I feared one of the major complications. I found the large craggy lump when I examined her abdomen. This malignancy was a well known complication of her condition but not all that common. Fate had been unkind to her. Again I think she knew. She didn't want to know the details and didn't ask.

I saw her often in the hospital as life sank slowly from her. She laughed and joked with those around her, obliterating their worries and lifting the spirits of the most depressed. She never spoke of her own problems. Patients loved to be with her and sought her out. Staff stayed overlong in her company. Her joy of life filled the place. She still spoke to everyone using foul four letter language. It didn't seem to matter.

One Monday morning I visited her and found she had little time left. She smiled at me.

'Doctor, how are you today?'

'I feel low on Mondays.'

I felt ashamed immediately as she looked at me with her fading but beautiful eyes, 'Oh Doctor, you mustn't feel like that. Don't you know that life is wonderful, so full of love and hope.'

When it appeared she had only one or two days left she asked a colleague about a coming show. He knew her need and brought to the hospital a dress, which in better times she would have modelled.

The nursing staff helped her into this extravagant beautiful gown. She died that night wearing it.

CHAPTER 8

The 25 Radiological Visiting Club

MANY HOSPITAL SPECIALTIES have visiting clubs whose members are selected from throughout Great Britain and Ireland. The purpose of these clubs in radiology is to meet, over a weekend, twice yearly to present papers on clinical subjects or research. Wives, husbands and partners of members are invited and a social programme is arranged for them. The list of members is small, to allow time for each member to make a contribution. Discussion is usually lively, analytical and instructive. The meetings provide an excellent forum for the exchange of views on clinical matters and as a testing ground for new ideas.

I belong to two such clubs, the younger of which is the Twenty Five Radiological Visiting Club, and the other, the Shadows Radiological Travelling Club. Each meets in spring and autumn. On the Saturday night of the weekend, a black tie dinner is held and on the Sunday the host entertains the club to lunch at his or her home. The membership of each is twenty five, but the number of emeritus members is increasing. Each member will host the meeting in rotation, and so the visits will move through the major centres of the country.

As one progresses up the consultant ladder, a mark of achievement is an invitation to join one of the clubs. An invitation to speak at a meeting is the preliminary step, followed by a period of anxiety waiting for the offer of membership which may or may not come. The clubs have an academic value but also foster long term friendships. I have enjoyed my membership of these two Radiological Clubs and have learnt much from the meetings. The quality of the presentations is high. Many times I returned home slightly depressed that my personal contribution and my ability were below the standards of my colleagues. This however spurred me to greater effort. I was also enriched by the quality of the clinical research presented by my colleagues. This also kept my teaching up to date. The contribution to the specialty of radiology made by the clubs is substantial and justifies credits given to their members for continuing medical education.

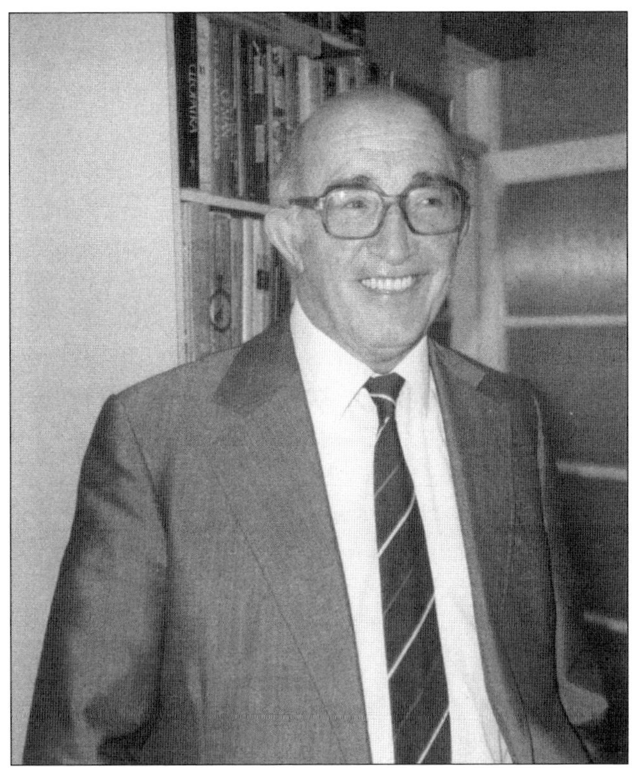

Dr Harold Issacson. Consultant Radiologist, Kings College Hospital, London

My first invitation came from the Twenty Five Radiological Visiting Club. I'm unaware who proposed my name but Dr Harold Isaacson mentioned the club to me early in my consultant career. Harold was older than me; an undergraduate prize winner, he graduated in medicine in Trinity College, Dublin in 1939. He specialized in clinical radiology studying at Bristol Royal Infirmary and The Royal Free Hospital following a long period as a general physician. Harold was an intelligent, conscientious doctor and an excellent radiologist. He was appointed consultant to King's College Hospital, Denmark Hill, London. His Russian Jewish parents had emigrated to Ireland. Dublin has a large Jewish community and their value in Dublin society is a model for others to copy. Jewish and Irish humour have much in common and Dublin is a fertile ground for humour. Harold however was a serious minded man, kind and concerned for his patients and indeed kind to junior colleagues or those in need of help. He was popular with the members of the club and enjoyed them sharing fun with him.

There was one memorable trip abroad. The club had been invited to a scientific meeting in Nurenburg, Germany in the 1960s. During the trip Harold wore a new trilby hat which was a source of pride to him. He forgot it when we left the plane and we waited while it was retrieved. A bus waited to take us to the hotel. Harold lost his hat which was found later above the seat he had initially taken but from which he had moved. Signing into the hotel he left his hat on the reception desk and one of the members found it. By this time Harold's hat was infamous. The corporate feeling was that to be rid of Harold's hat would be a joy. However Harold's hat was to be further distinguished on this trip. A few nights after we arrived after some days of excellent clinical discussions, the members and their wives went to a restaurant for a gourmet meal. I remember the night clearly and can still see the rows of wine bottles which as they were emptied were placed against the wall behind the table. I couldn't believe we could drink so much. If one doesn't drink often, an excess can be devastating and that was the only time I've ever seen Harold out of control. Being in a restaurant known for its good food, the clientele were quiet and bent to their chosen sport in a studied manner. To eat good food was for them a serious sport. Our large table was not so quiet and this distraction to the other diners was noticeable and getting worse by the bottle. Harold's voice was getting louder and his Jewish origin becoming more and more a matter of pride to him in these Nurenburg surroundings with all its history. Things may not have got worse if Harold hadn't burst into song. Even his loud and poor singing might have been tolerated, but when he choose to sing 'It's a long way to Tipperary', shouts of protest erupted from the Germans all over the restaurant. Quickly the proprietors ushered us out, handing our coats to us at the door. We staggered back to the hotel carefully controlling Harold. When we got to the hotel there was consternation. Harold's hat was still at the restaurant. We restrained him from going back for it. We thought the night had ended successfully and we loved Harold even more. Harold bought a toy gun for his son. It looked remarkably real and was confiscated at the airport.

Colonel Desmond Whyte was a member of the Twenty Five Club. He was the bravest man I've ever known and the most humble of the great men I've known.

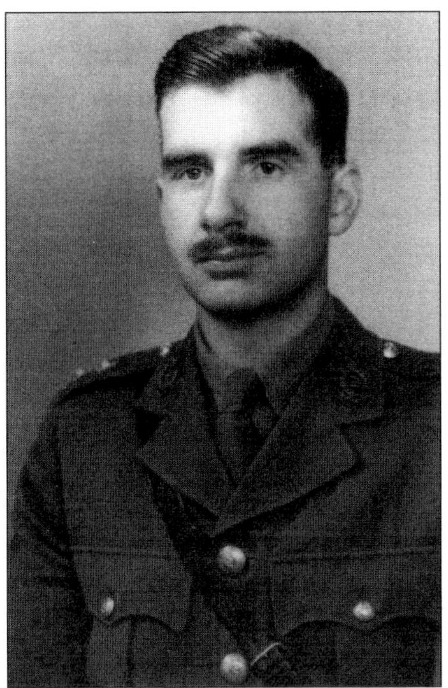

Colonel Desmond Whyte DSO. Consultant Radiologist Altnagelvin Hospital, Londonderry, Northern Ireland

Desmond Gilbert Cromie Whyte was born in Belfast in 1913. He qualified in medicine in Queen's University, Belfast in 1937. Following the usual house officer posts he joined the Royal Army Medical Corps in 1939 and was Regimental Medical Officer with the Worcestershire Regiment. He next served with PIA Force (Persia and Iraq) and in 1944 was appointed Commanding Officer of the 11th Indian Field Ambulance in 111 Brigade commanded by John Masters, the author. About his war service I can do no better than quote extracts from Desmond's obituary. I don't know who wrote it. Desmond was a Chindit, a member of the force created by Orde Wingate, designed to destroy the Japanese reputation of invincibility in the jungle during World War Two. Desmond flew into the Burmese jungle with the second expedition in 1944, behind the Japanese lines. The Chindits destroyed Japanese instillations and inflicted heavy casualties. After a month expecting to be withdrawn they were told to move north and divert the Japanese from attacks carried out by General Stillwell's troops. The Japanese attacked, determined to destroy the Chindits. Rain fell continously and the Chindits were plagued by malaria, dysentery, insects, leeches and all manner of war wounds. Desmond Whyte had many narrow escapes, but cared for the wounded, the sick and the dying and despite the shell fire all around him oversaw the movement of one hundred and eighty of these victims over eighteen miles of mud. Although wounded himself he saved at least two hundred others. He was always ready with cheerful wisdom, always whistling something sentimental and always out of tune. He had the engaging knack of encouraging a man beyond his strength when the occasion demanded it.

He described the Japanese as utterly ruthless and without compassion. 'I found a friend pinioned to a teak tree with a bayonet through both the left and right wrist; and the lower limbs missing, eaten by hungry jackals. The aim was to make us so terrified that we would wish not to continue fighting. It had the opposite effect.'

I'll quote an extract from *Chindit* by Richard Rhodes James.

'I arrived with tattered feet and presented myself to the Medical Officer, Major Whyte. He had just arrived and I had the first glimpse of a remarkable man, tireless, fearless and infinitely reassuring in time of trouble. It is a pity that we could not think of any more significant name for him than "Doc".'

Further evidence of the unique qualities of Desmond Whyte are these extracts from *The Road past Mandalay*, by John Masters.

'Desmond Whyte, half naked, soft voiced with the Ulster brogue, kept at his work day and night, as he already had for a hundred days and a hundred nights. I write out another Victoria Cross citation, this time for a man who above all others, has kept the brigade going – Desmond Whyte. (It is supported by my four battalion commanders, but Desmond has not dashed out and rescued one wounded man under fire, he has only saved two hundred over a hundred days, calm, efficient and cheerful while shells blast the bodies to pieces under his hands. The Cross is refused and he gets the Distinguished Service Order instead. This is not good enough.)'

Colonel Desmond Whyte retired from the army in 1957. He studied radiology at St Mary's Hospital in London and was appointed Consultant Radiologist to Altnagelvin Hospital in Londonderry, Northern Ireland. While there he set up a school of radiography and trained many radiographers with the help of colleague radiologists. A Knight of St John, a Justice of the Peace, he was Chairman of the Northern

Ireland Cancer Research Campaign and became High Sheriff of Londonderry.

When I hosted a meeting of the Twenty Five Club in London, at lunch in my home, Desmond met Ronald Brown, a fellow Chindit, for the first time since they both served in Burma. It was an emotional moment.

I consider it an honour to have been a close friend of Desmond Whyte.

Desmond Hawkins is another member of the Twenty Five Club. His family came from Cork in Southern Ireland. Desmond qualified in medicine at St Mary's Hospital Medical School, and after taking his Membership of the Royal College of Physicians specialized in radiology. His main interest was in neurological disease and he became President of the British Society of Neuroradiology. His national service was spent in the Royal Air Force and his consultant appointment was to Addenbrooke's Hospital in Cambridge.

Desmond had an interest in teaching and training and was appointed Dean of the School of Clinical Medicine of Cambridge. In addition to academic excellence he had manual skills. At a time when it was surgically difficult or sometimes impossible to treat certain disorders of the vascular circulation of the brain which threatened life, Desmond manipulated catheters through the major arteries of the head and neck to the site of the blood vessel weakness. Under direct vision, using radiological imaging he repaired the damaged blood vessels. He performed these delicate procedures in Addenbrooke's Hospital in Cambridge but his reputation was national and international. His advice was sought from near and far. His work demanded a strong calm mind, a steady hand and critical judgement. He made a significant contribution to radiology and is held in esteem by his medical colleagues.

In retirement Desmond became President of Hughes Hall Cambridge. He also studied archaeology and wrote a book of scholarship entitled, *The Drainage of Wilbraham, Fulbourn and Feversham Fens*. The text illustrates how the drainage dictated the type and quality of the farming in this area of England.

Max Ryan, a founder member of the Twenty Five Radiological Visiting Club, qualified in the medical school of the Royal College of Surgeons in Ireland. I was a student demonstrator in Anatomy when he began his studies. Little did I know we would be professionally close in

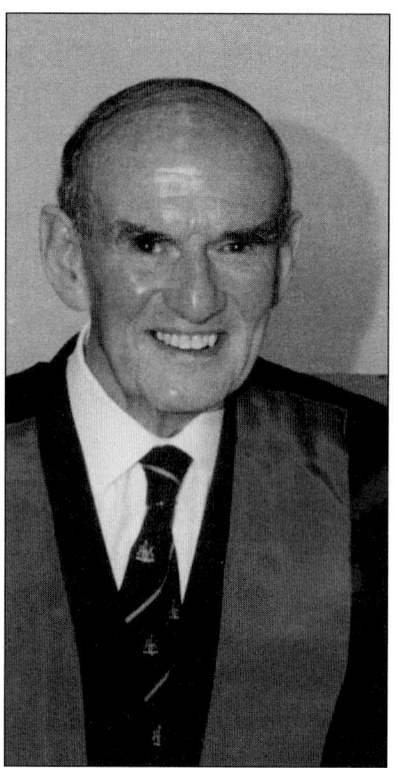

Professor Max Ryan. Consultant Radiologist. Past Dean Faculty of Radiologists, Royal College of Surgeons, Ireland

later years. Max has a wonderful sense of humour and as a student mirrored the carefree, bohemian fun-loving role attributed to Dublin students. He and a group of friends drove a lovely old convertible car, similar to that seen in the films of the 'Keystone Cops'. When one of the boys was taking out a girlfriend, another would put on a chauffeur's hat and drive him to pick her up.

This was very impressive.

Having qualified Max studied Radiology in Manchester. He was appointed consultant to the Richmond Hospital in Dublin. His application to his chosen specialty was total and he kept abreast of radiological advances to the benefit of his patients and his hospital, earning the respect of both. He became a lecturer and then Professor in the Royal College of Surgeons in Ireland and an examiner for the Fellowship of the Faculty of Radiology. He was elected Dean of the Faculty which he served with distinction.

In 1973 Max invited me to speak at the 43rd Inaugural Meeting of the Biological Society of the College (I had been a member of the Society as a student). That year Max was President-Elect of the Society. A fellow speaker was Professor Howard Middlemiss from Bristol. Max met Nancy and me at the airport and we stayed at his home just outside Dublin. On the way to the College that night Max said, 'The President is coming to the meeting.'

'What President? The President of the College?'

'No, Erskine Childers, the President of Ireland.'

'You can't be serious, Max.'

'Yes I am. You'll see.'

As we approached the College, the roads around had been closed for the approach of the President. I was surprised and still am that the President of Ireland would attend a meeting of the Biological Society of the Royal College of Surgeons. When I put this to Max his reply was,

'He's interested in medicine.'

A formal dinner was held at 7.00 p.m. when the President, his Aide de Camp and entourage, including the Chief of Police, arrived. Nancy and I along with Howard Middlemiss were introduced to the President. At the excellent dinner much wine was taken. At 8.00 p.m. we adorned ourselves with academic gowns and preceded by the College mace and the President we paraded into the lecture theatre. The audience, all in evening dress, rose. The formality of the occasion pleased me. I love the pomp.

Max and Howard spoke before me. When I rose to speak I felt a tinge of pride that I was speaking in the presence of the President of Ireland. A few minutes into the lecture I looked to the front seats, full of my own importance, to see the President.

He was asleep. I felt deflated and thought this may have been his opinion of my worth. I carried on regardless.

Following further speeches we paraded out at 10.00 p.m. I was walking beside Max who said, 'Now, we have a party.'

The audience went to one room and the President, his entourage and the speakers to another, with a dividing door between. We drank and chatted. Max, the President-Elect, presented me with a book of the history of the Royal College of Surgeons in Ireland which the President of Ireland signed. At 11.00 p.m. the President retired and the dividing doors were opened and the audience joined us. There was more wine, chatter and laughter. Friends sought each other all over the large room. Alcohol and time began to tell and I looked for Nancy.

'I'm tired.'

She replied, 'I'm exhausted, but we can't leave.'

Max was full of energy, moving about the room, laughing, shaking hands, making introductions and clapping backs. He came to us again about midnight.

'I think we should leave soon. I've a party starting at home after this.'

'My God, Max we're nearly dead.'

'Ah, sure the night's young and your plane isn't until later in the day.'

We staggered out of the College into the car and followed by a cavalcade headed for the outskirts of Dublin. Car after car drove up to Max's home. Bottles of wine were opened and the chat, the stories and the music began.

At about 3.00 a.m. I said to Max,

'I can't take any more – of anything. We're going to bed.'

As I lay in bed I could hear the thump of the music and the laughter. I then lost conciousness.

At 8.00 a.m. Max appeared with our breakfast on a tray.

'Max, you're wearing jodpurs.'

'Yes, I've been riding.'

At 10.30 a.m. we went downstairs.

'Would you like a drink?'

'If I have a drink it'll kill me.'

Max replied,

'If I don't have a drink it'll kill me.'

I can't remember getting the plane home, but we did.

Apart from his contribution to general and specialized radiology, Max is an acknowledged expert on the medico-legal aspects of radiology. He is a member of the Medical Protection Society and is consulted frequently as an expert witness in Irish cases of litigation. He is an Honorary Fellow of the American College of Radiologists and has written extensively. Max has taught radiology in Kuwait, examined in Baghdad and advised in Saudi Arabia.

The Royal College of Radiologists of the United Kingdom held two joint meetings with the Faculty in Ireland in recent years. They were most successful educationally and in addition were social gatherings of extraordinary popularity. At one of these meetings a reception was held in Dublin Castle, a beautifully preserved building furnished in exquisite taste. At that event whiskey and gin circulated in Waterford glass jugs.

The last combined meeting I attended in Dublin was when I was President of the Royal College of Radiologists. It too was a great academic and social success.

I was pleased that Max represented radiology in Ireland having been Dean of the Faculty in Ireland and I represented British radiology and we had both qualified in medicine from the same medical school in Dublin.

Max had his share of problems. When young he developed poliomyelitis from which he made a good recovery. In adult life he had acute gall bladder disease complicated by septicaemia and was seriously ill. He has had several acute episodes to which less robust men would have succumbed. His survival owes much to his strength of character. His strength of character owes much to his strong Catholic faith which I admire so much. His sense of fun is contagious. While abroad with members of the Twenty Five Club we stayed in a small hotel in Germany. The reception clerk was an elderly man, a hunchback who walked with a tilt to one side with a loose hanging arm, not unlike the hunchback of Notre Dame. He was bad tempered and spoke with heavily accented English. When we returned late in the evening he wasn't behind the reception desk. We waited quite a while but eventually Max went behind the desk, adopted the stance of the reception clerk and said to each of us in turn.

'Vat eis ze noomber of ze rim?'

This was met with howls of laughter as he handed us our keys. We turned to see the reception clerk watching us from the doorway. We hurried to bed very embarrassed. None of us, including Max, wished our humour to be hurtful. Without humour in our medical lives we would perish.

Other members of the Twenty Five Club whom I hold in great affection include Peter Phelps, who had an international reputation in the radiology of ear, nose and throat disease, Myles McNulty, consultant in Bath and an oarsman whom I met every year at Henley Regatta until his death some years ago, Bob Verney, consultant in Cambridge with whom I examined for the Fellowship in Hong Kong, Ken Rowley, consultant in Blackpool who worked tirelessly single handed, Norman

Lewtas, a neuroradiologist in Sheffield, who died some years ago, and was the epitome of an English gentleman. My generation have either passed on or are emeritus and a new membership is in existence. I still go the meetings but radiology has advanced so much in recent decades that I feel like a dinosaur.

Chapter 9

The Shadows

The senior of the two Radiological Travelling Clubs to which I belong is 'The Shadows'. Like the Twenty Five Club the members are confined to twenty five in number chosen from throughout the United Kingdom. I don't know who proposed me but I well remember my first meeting which was held in a hotel close by Lake Windermere. Ian Kerr, a radiological consultant from the Brompton Hospital, and a close friend, is a member. He suggested Nancy and I should travel to Lake Windermere with him and his wife Nesta. On Friday we travelled by train to Carlisle where a hired car was waiting. We then drove through winding roads to the banks of the lake which seemed to stretch for miles and in the falling darkness was haunting.

Most of the members of The Shadows were senior to me and I was delighted that Professor Robert Steiner and Dr John Laws were members. Robert and John were the radiologists in the Hammersmith Hospital who had impressed me so much and influenced me in my future career. Now some years later I was a guest at the club, anticipating an invitation to be a member. This depended on the quality of my clinical presentation at the scientific meeting on Saturday, and my overall acceptability as a colleague. I was apprehensive. Considering the events of the weekend I was thankful that the invitation came. As in the Twenty Five Club there is a formal dinner on the Saturday night. On that first visit I met a legendary radiologist, Dr Reggie Reid from Manchester. He was a neuroradiologist, a renowned teacher and a larger than life character. At the end of dinner in this club the ceremony of the Loving Cup is held where the silver cup is filled with champagne and circulated round the members and their wives in the age-old fashion of such ceremonies. Three members stand at a time and the one drinking is protected by another standing at his or her back while facing the one in front who then receives the cup and so on around the room. The cup has added value in that it has engraved on it, since the inception of the club, the signatures of all the members. The host for the evening is responsible for the cup and I regret to say that on one

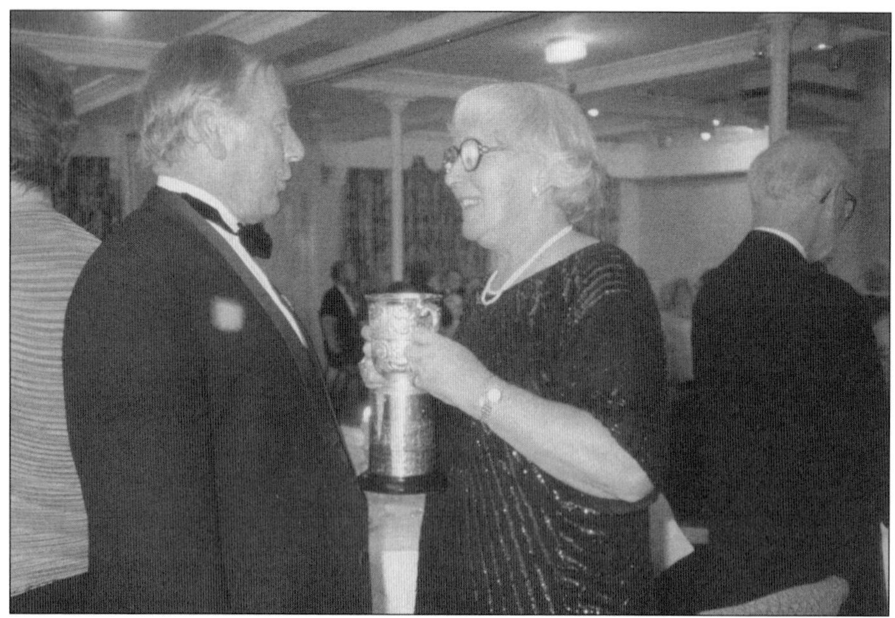

The author and Nancy performing the ceremony of the loving cup

occasion when I hosted the meeting at a hotel in Surrey, I left it on the dining table and went to bed.

In the morning my telephone rang, 'Ian here, Oscar, have you lost something.'

'No, not that I know.'

'Think hard. Have you mislaid something very valuable?'

'No, Nancy is here.'

'Very funny, but have you forgotten a valuable piece of silver?'

'My God, Ian. Where is the loving cup?'

'You left it on the table, but relax, I've got it.'

'Thank God, Ian.'

'No, thank me, Oscar.'

On this first visit after the loving cup had been passed around all the members retired to an adjoining room for more drinks. There was a piano at one end and to my surprise Reggie Reid began to play music hall tunes with great gusto and expertise. Even more to my surprise I stood by the piano and sang the songs. Robert Steiner is game for anything and joined me. We sang together for almost an hour. All the wives were astonished but the fun of the evening was only beginning.

Reggie had an unusual sharp and bizarre sense of humour which matched my own, and the singing was followed by hilarious jokes and antics. This was not the usual outcome of these evenings, but later I was told that on a previous occasion, Reggie who had more than his usual share of wine, had disappeared. A search was organized and he was found asleep in the wrong room, on the wrong floor, in the empty bed of an unknown hotel guest, who fortunately hadn't returned at the time. He was taken to his own room by his colleagues as quickly and quietly as possible. On this my first night with this club, everyone made sure Reggie got to the right bed. Reggie was a smoker and suffered from bronchitis. Shortly after this meeting when on holiday in the West Indies, sugarcane fields were being burnt and Reggie was overexposed to the fumes. He died.

That weekend with The Shadows was the only time I met him, although I'd known his reputation for years. I regret I hadn't met him earlier. We haven't had hilarious evenings quite like that ever since. Perhaps it's just as well.

The Shadows Radiological Travelling Club is another excellent forum for presenting clinical cases and research. The clinical meeting occupies all Saturday which ends with the formal dinner. The evaluation of the members clinical presentation is helpful, both to us as doctors and eventually to our patients. The audience is critical but constructive. As with the Twenty Five Club I came home more despondent than ever about the quality of my own work. Most of the members were so senior that I would have to work hard to reach their standard.

Many of the members have held academic posts in the College. Among the Presidents of the College were Sir Thomas Lodge, Sir Howard Middlemiss, Professor Robert Steiner, Dr John Laws, Professor Peter Armstrong and myself. Members who were Vice-Presidents were Dr Ian Kerr and Dr Dennis Stoker. Many of these members at varying times held other posts in the College such as editors and wardens. All the members have clinical and teaching posts in prestigious hospitals known for their high academic standards. Regretfully Tommy, Howard and John have died, but the remainder of those I have mentioned still attend the meetings and watch with pleasure the continuing progress of our younger colleagues.

One of the best academic radiologists in the United Kingdom I have known is Professor Robert Steiner. Robert was born in Prague in 1918.

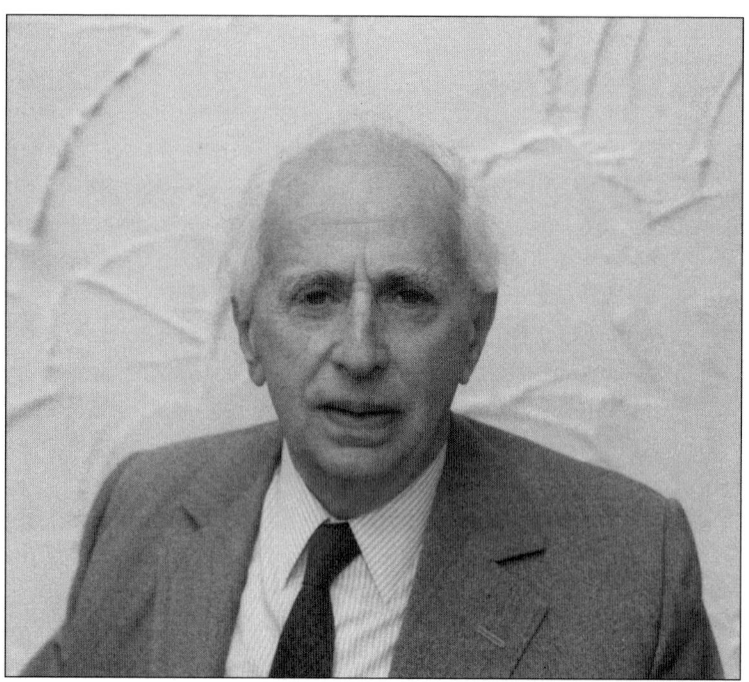

Professor Robert Steiner. Professor of Radiology, Hammersmith Hospital and Post Graduate Medical School. Past President Royal College of Radiologists

He received his primary education in Vienna and influenced by the medical family into which his sister had married, decided, when aged fifteen, to study medicine. He entered the University of Vienna in 1935 and completed his pre-clinical studies in 1938. When Hitler and the German Army entered Vienna in 1938, Robert had to leave and an anxious search was made for a suitable country and medical school in which he could finish his studies. The advice was to go to the British Isles. At the time Robert had an older brother, a chemical physicist in Cambridge. Robert came to England and applied to London University. The university would not recognize his pre-clinical years in Vienna and he would have to start at the beginning again. This would prove to be a great burden in time and finance. He decided to try the University of Edinburgh who gave the same decision, and next the University of Belfast with similar results. Then he wrote to the University of Ireland in Dublin. They expressed interest in his years of pre-clinical study in Vienna which they considered an excellent medical school, and were prepared to permit Robert to enter the clinical school. Robert sailed for Dublin and began his clinical studies in October 1938, attending the Richmond Hospital. Until then his studies had been in his native tongue, but now they had to be completed reading, writing and speaking in English. There was the additional problem of understanding the Irish brogue. This cannot have been easy. During his time at the Richmond hospital, influenced by the surgeons, he had leanings to specialize in surgery. On qualifying in 1941 he describes his feelings as one of great relief and happiness. This didn't last long as in the face of native Irish competition and too many graduates he was unable to get a house physician's job,which is essential for further progress in medicine. Aware of the seriousness of his situation he thought the only chance of a house post was in the United Kingdom. A further serious problem arose. The war was in progress and Robert had no nationality. Austria no longer existed and he didn't have a German passport. He was in effect stateless. He tried to join the British Armed Forces but was not permitted to do so, being classified as an alien. He contacted a friend, Dr Hajiek, who had taught many British surgeons, and got a letter of introduction to the senior Ear, Nose and Throat surgeon in Guy's Hospital in London. Helped by the British Medical Association, who were aware of the need for doctors, and the Guy's surgeon, Robert got an introduction to the head of the Emergency Medical Service (EMS). This led to a post in Guy's Hospital. This was six months after qualifying. The EMS sent doctors where the need was greatest and Robert was sent to do house posts in medicine and surgery in Macclesfield until 1942.

Next he did orthopaedics in Winnick in a 1000-bedded hospital under the consultancy of Mr Barnes who later became Professor of Orthopaedics in Glasgow. It was here that a major influence came into Robert's life. The radiologist at Winnick was Dr George Chance, an Irishman, who became a close friend. He persuaded Robert that a career in radiology was a realistic ambition and one he should pursue. Robert, who had never contemplated radiology as a future specialty, watched George Chance at work and understood for the first time its complexity and fascination.

Dr A.B. Barclay in 1944 was recruiting trainees for radiology on behalf of the EMS. Robert applied and was accepted. He was posted to Sheffield. This was a busy time, working six days a week and visiting hospitals in Chesterfield, Barnsley and Scunthorpe. During this time he was receiving personal tuition from senior radiologists. Dr Thomas Lodge, who was to become a personal friend and colleague, was senior assistant in Sheffield and gave Robert enormous support. (Tommy Lodge became President of the Faculty of Radiology in 1963.) Robert took the Diploma in Radiology in 1945 and the Fellowship of the Faculty in 1948. A thesis was then part of the examination and Tommy Lodge had done his on the pulmonary circulation while Robert worked with him, and this influenced his own future work.

In 1950 Robert was appointed Deputy Director and Lecturer in Diagnostic Radiology at the Hammersmith Hospital. In 1957 he became Director and in 1960 was appointed Professor of Diagnostic Radiology, University of London, in the Hammersmith Hospital and the Postgraduate Medical School of London.

Robert's career has been one of acknowledged excellence and his influence on radiology in the United Kingdom and internationally has been outstanding. He holds the Fellowships of the major British medical Royal Colleges and the Honorary Fellowships of the American College of Radiology, the Australasian College, the Faculty of Radiology in Ireland and the Academy of Medicine in Singapore. He is an honorary Member of the Radiological Society of North America (RSNA) and numerous European Societies. He was President of the British Institute of Radiology in 1972 and held numerous posts in the Faculty of Radiologists. The Royal College of Radiologists was established in 1975 and Howard Middlemiss was its first President, Robert followed from 1977 until 1980. He was awarded the Barclay Medal in 1961, made a Companion of the British Empire (CBE) in 1979 and awarded the Gold Medal of the Royal College of Radiologists in 1985. He has published over 250 scientific papers in chest and cardiovascular subjects and in later years Magnetic Resonance Imaging (MRI).

In 1983 in a publication of Recent Advances in Radiology and Medical Imaging a large number of distinguished radiologists wrote, 'We would like this volume to mark Robert Steiner's fourth decade in academic radiology. His outstanding achievement needs no further comment.' Robert is a kind, concerned man who holds his fellow man in high regard, and demands of himself and others a high standard of moral and professional behaviour. My friendship with Robert has grown over the years and today I feel privileged to have that friendship which is beyond price. In Gertie, his wife, he has the perfect companion and mentor. They have befriended many medical men and women throughout their lives and are looked up to as an example hard to follow.

There were some memorable meetings of 'The Shadows'. When Dr John Tudor of Addenbrooke's Hospital, Cambridge was the host, the meeting was held in a hotel in Lavenham. I came home from St Mary's Hospital on Friday evening and Nancy and I set off for Suffolk in a torrent of rain. Within an hour, this became a storm of frightening severity. I had difficulty seeing the road, so fierce was the wind and rain. Off the motorway we had to navigate through deep rivers of water. I cannot remember why, but we were in Nancy's car, a Volkswagen Golf, and in the middle of one 'pond', the car stopped. I couldn't get it started, no doubt due to the engine being drenched in water. I tried time and time again, but worried that the battery would run down.

'Darling, could you start the engine, if I got out and pushed?'

'How do I do that?'

'You put it into second gear and when the speed picks up, let out the clutch, then when the engine fires, accelerate.'

'Can't you do that?'

'If I do, you have to get out and push.'

'I'd rather do that.'

'Are you sure?'

'Yes.'

It was pouring with rain. Nancy is a strong woman. She pushed, the car started. We navigated more 'ponds' and the car stopped three times. We wondered about our sanity, but to turn back would have been equally problematical. As we approached Lavenham, a policeman in high gum boots, stopped us. 'Good evening, sir, there's a large pool of water here which is very deep on both sides.'

'What do you think I should do?

'I've been guiding cars through and if you follow me you'll get past.'

He walked in front, obviously trusting I wouldn't run him down. We got through with the engine still running.

'Thank you, Officer.'

'It's a pleasure, sir.'

This was one occasion when the approach of a policeman to my car wasn't ominous. We arrived at the hotel exhausted and wet through. At least Nancy was.

'The first thing I need is a drink.'

Nancy replied, 'Me too.'

The scientific meeting started the next morning and following the morning session we met the ladies for lunch. Prawns were on the menu. I'm allergic to shell fish, but Nancy loves them. She was conditioned following the previous night to indulge herself and she had a hefty helping.

The afternoon scientific session went well, and we retired to our rooms to change for dinner.

'Oscar, I feel a little ill. I've got some stomach ache and feel a bit sick.'

'You've had too much excitement and pushing that car was a bad idea. You'll feel better when you've had a bath and are changed for dinner.'

We went downstairs to the pre-dinner reception.

'Oscar, I can't stand. I must sit down, I feel ill.'

'Sit for a while. I'm sure you'll be alright.'

After a few minutes, 'I'm going to vomit, I can't go in to dinner. I'm going to bed.' She did both – went to bed and vomited. She didn't get to the dinner.

I went ahead, and during the dinner three ladies and one man left to go to bed feeling ill. Prawns!

When it was my turn to host the shadows, I booked the Burford Bridge Hotel, Box Hill. I sent out the invitations, the scientific and the social programmes in good time many months beforehand. It was to be an unusual weekend as, for the first time, we were going to include an exhibition of arts and crafts, the hobbies of the members and their wives. This required some detailed planning.

About a month before the meeting I had a telephone call.

'This is the Facilities Manager of the Burford Bridge Hotel. Dr Craig can I come to see you?'

'Why's that?'

'I need to talk to you about your meeting of The Shadows.'

'Can't we do it on the phone?'

'No, I must see you.'

This caused me some anxiety and I made an appointment. A lady and a gentleman came to my home.

'Dr Craig, we know that you booked the hotel for The Shadows twelve months ago, but there has been a problem.'

'What's that?'

'The booking "fell off" the computer and we've booked a wedding reception for the same time.'

'My God, I've sent out all the details, all the instructions to all the members some time ago.'

'We will honour our obligation to you as you booked first, but I must tell you that the bride's mother is having hysterics and is threatening to kill herself. Can we suggest an alternative solution?'

'What's that?

'We have another hotel, Ghyll Manor in Rusper. It's smaller, but can hold your group. It's a lovely venue and you can have it for the price we've already agreed'

'Gosh, I don't know.'

'Would you please come and see Ghyll Manor?'

'Yes, I'll do that.'

We all drove out to Ghyll Manor. It was lovely and in many ways more attractive than Burford Bridge for our purposes. We would take over the whole manor except for one room. The facilities for the scientific session were excellent and there was a suitable room for the Arts and Crafts exhibition. They promised to notify the members of the change of venue for me, if I agreed. The only small problem was the longer drive to my home for the lunch on the Sunday. I couldn't complain. I agreed.

The weekend was an enormous success and I was well pleased with the management of the Burford Bridge Hotel. In addition we may have saved a suicide!

The Arts and Crafts exhibition was also a success. Dr Gryspeedt showed his silver work, John Laws his sculpture. John had only studied sculpture in retirement and already had done the heads of four Presidents of the Royal College of Radiologists: Sir Thomas Lodge, Professors Robert Steiner, Rhys Davies and myself. They are in the College now. There were a few artists, Ian Lavelle, Geraint Roberts, Diana Laws and Nancy. Uschi Kellet also showed her sculpture, Jennie Simpkins a dress she had made designed from the stars and planets, Jill Guyer her pottery. I exhibited two poems suitably framed. To date we've only had two Hobbies Exhibitions at our meetings. Maybe we should have more.

There was an unusual meeting of the Twenty Five Club. It was to be held in Belfast, hosted by Colonel Desmond Whyte. Many younger members were reluctant to go to Northern Ireland as there was so much terrorism going on, and their wives said that because of their young children they should miss this one. However a sizeable number did gather at Heathrow. We boarded the plane. Surprisingly almost all the elder members were in the front where most of the subsequent action took place.

While sitting on the runway at 8.30 a.m. the captain spoke, 'Ladies and Gentlemen, this is the captain speaking.' That always makes my heart sink.

'We have a minor problem and I will be returning to our stand to have it sorted out.'

The plane returned but we didn't care for this development and were not without some anxiety.

A cabin staff announcement followed.

'Ladies and Gentlemen, we will serve drinks by courtesy of British Airways.'

This surprised us, at this time in the morning and sitting in the plane on the stand. We were served with double whiskies and double gins. We sat and chatted and shortly we laughed. The noise level began to rise. At 9.30 a.m. another round of drinks was served, and again doubles. We elder members in the front were now making merry with jokes flying around the cabin, laughter hitting the ceiling and no sense of anxiety to be found. At 10.30 a.m. another double round appeared. At this stage we thought we could fly to Ireland without the plane. If we never got off the ground we thought we'd had a successful meeting and were quite happy about it.

Sometime after 11.00 a.m. Desmond Hawkins said to an air hostess, 'We could get off and board the 12.00 o'clock shuttle.'

'Sir, we are the 12.00 o'clock shuttle.'

We cannot remember taking off or landing. But we did. I would recommend this treatment for all air flights.

Chapter 10

Some Characters of St Mary's Hospital and Medical School

There were twelve teaching hospitals in London. A teaching hospital is one with an undergraduate medical school. The London teaching hospitals and medical schools were St Bartholomew's, Guy's, St Thomas's, The Royal London. The Royal Free, Middlesex, Charing Cross, Westminster, St Mary's, University College, St George's and Kings.

Each medical school has a strong sense of identity, a long tradition and, like soldiers in army regiments such as the Guards, each student has a pride of association. Each medical school has played a part in the development of medicine and illustrious medical names are associated with each. We all like to think that our own medical school leads the field in excellence and accordingly the rivalry is strong. We each like to score in debate and conversation regarding another. Many times I've said, 'he qualified in Bart's but is a good man none the less.' Another is, 'he's a Charing Cross man, but despite this has done remarkably well.' These remarks, said in jest, are accepted as typical of medical school humour. It's difficult however to convey the strong sense of pride that is part of being a Bart's man or woman, or a Guy's man or woman or a graduate of any of the London medical schools. Along with this pride comes an arrogance. This arrogance of belonging to a London medical school is poison to those qualified elsewhere. The truth is that the quality of medical teaching and the excellence of the medical schools in the United Kingdom differs little if at all from place to place, and the excellence or otherwise of the graduate is dependent on him or her and not the school. However there is good to be had from the vanity associated with each. My medical school was the school of the Royal College of Surgeons in Ireland.

It was when I came to St Mary's Hospital in London in 1957 that I developed pride in the hospital and medical school, where I became the Director of Clinical Studies. Being in practice there for thirty five years,

I identify totally with St Mary's and I too have the arrogance of association with this London based teaching hospital. There are advantages to appointment as a consultant in a teaching hospital, as the teaching of medical students and young postgraduates is part of everyday practice. This keeps each consultant up to date and alert to changing ideas and methods. Lecturing is part of medical school life, as is the publishing of academic and clinical papers. Thus there is a sharp edge to daily practice and one is exposed to colleagues who can be critical of another's ability both clinically and academically. This is no bad thing and is part of 'the buzz' of teaching hospital practice.

The rivalry between the teaching hospitals is not confined to clinical or academic excellence but extends to sports. The sports are varied and include water polo, hockey, cricket, fencing, rowing, sailing and football among others, but perhaps the most competitive is seen on the rugby field. St Mary's Hospital Medical School had a reputation for favouring rugby playing students. There was much truth in this in the past. The hospital was opened in 1851, the medical school in 1854 and the St Mary's Hospital Rugby Football Club founded in 1865. The tradition St Mary's had for rugby was fostered by 'the great Dean', Dr Charles Wilson, later Sir Charles and later still Lord Moran. He became Sir Winston Churchill's doctor and wrote a controversial book about his time with him. He also became President of the Royal College of Physicians and played some part in the formation of the National Health Service after the war. Lord Moran guided the medical school through difficult times in the early years of the 20th century and raised much-needed capital. He established Professorial clinical units. He awarded Rugby Scholarships to selected young men to study medicine. He was convinced that the qualities that made a good rugby player were those that made a good doctor. He wanted men of character as well as academic ability. These qualities included the ability to work with a team, to face adversity or even defeat and continue the fray. These qualities are reminiscent of Kipling's 'if you can keep your head when all about you' etc. He also believed that these were the qualities encouraged in the best British public schools, which he visited in search of candidates. He and only he chose whom he wished to admit.

The tradition for rugby players at St Mary's continued until recently and St Mary's has won the Hospital Rugby Cup more than any other London medical school, passing the record held by Guy's some years

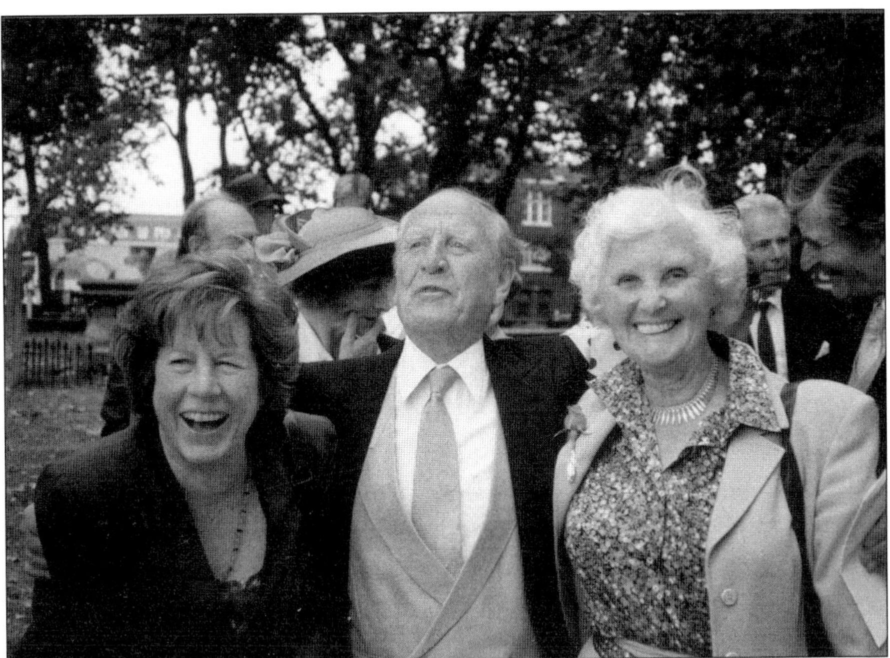

Dr Binine Williams, Dr Harold Edwards, Past Dean of St Mary's Hospital Medical School, Lady Peart (Wife of Sir Stanley Peart) (Left to right)

ago. There was however no sacrifice of academic achievement. Future Deans placed less emphasis on rugby and other attributes, such as proficiency in music, were to become important. There was still an emphasis on extra curricular skills as well as academic achievement and St Mary's has a thriving Dramatic Society, a worthy Music Society, an excellent choir, a great orchestra and an exciting jazz band in addition to a multitude of sporting activities.

The competition to get a consultant post in any teaching hospital was keen. I think this was especially so in London, but is changing. The price of property in the capital is such that few can afford to live close to their teaching hospital and the hassle of commuting is unwelcome. To go by car is extremely tedious and time wasting, to travel by public transport is a nightmare. Who would wish to rear children in the centre of London or its environs? Fewer graduates wish to join this 'rat race', but the totally committed still apply.

I never thought I had the necessary qualities to apply for a London teaching hospital post, but circumstances drove me there. I have loved every minute of my work at St Mary's. I have loved my association with the students and postgraduates and with the medical school. Like many of my colleagues there is more than a little of the 'prima donna' in my makeup. With few exceptions my colleagues have been wonderful and I've appreciated and been stimulated by their eccentricities and skills. I've made life-long friends.

I've written elsewhere about my friendship with Dr Harold Edwards, consultant neurologist and dean of St Mary's Medical School. He too became a St Mary's man although he qualified in Guy's. We were friends for all my time at St Mary's. I followed Harold as Director of Clinical Studies in 1968. We shared a love of rugby and attended international matches together. We shared a love of cars. Together with our wives we dined at home and in favourite restaurants frequently. We holidayed together at home and abroad. Harold and I had similar attitudes to our work and to our colleagues. He was older than me and I learnt much from him about life. He was an astute observer of human behaviour and a rigidly self disciplined man.

We also shared a sense of humour although differing in many ways. We appeared on stage in the medical school and our yearly performance in a sketch when we soaked each other with the contents of a soda siphon was repeatedly requested by the students. Harold was a superb clinician and his neurology was based on the age-old skills of clinical history taking and analysis and immaculate clinical examination. When technology advanced he embraced the advantages of radiological scanning but never lost sight of the persona and the mind of the patient that could not be assessed by technological aids. He was meticulous in his dedication to the National Health Service and never gave short measure with his time or his attention to patients. If students fell short of his expectations his tolerance was limited, but his behaviour as a consultant and his attitude to patients was a worthy example to those he taught. Harold died some years ago, and I still miss him and his wisdom.

A dear friend is Professor Sir Stanley Peart, FRS. He is an extraordinary man, flamboyant, bow-tied and extrovert. Stan is a gifted academic with the bedside touch of a down to earth family doctor. He is kind, concerned and conscientious. His original work on the relationship of kidney disease to high blood pressure and his overall reputation in research earned him his Knighthood and his Fellowship of the Royal Society. He was schooled at King's College School,

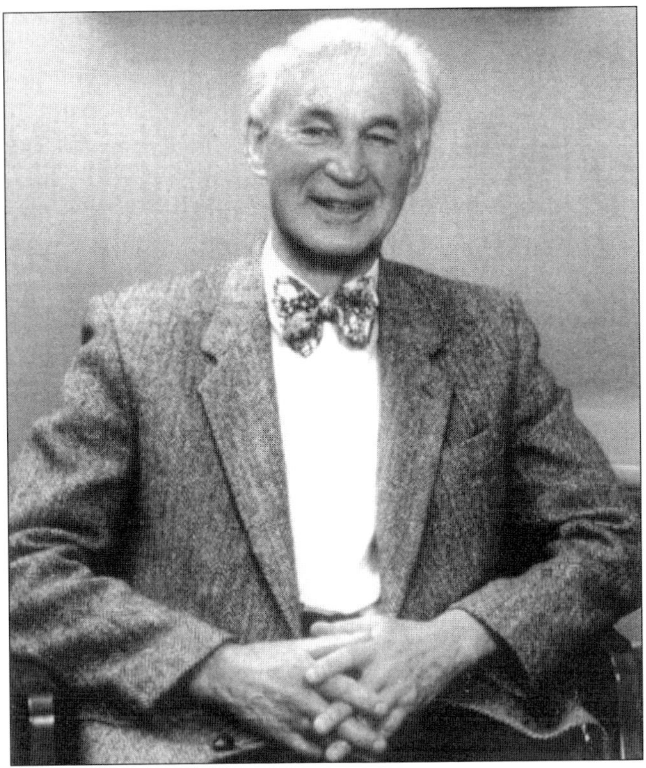

Sir Stanley Peart. Professor of Medicine, St Mary's Hospital Medical School, University of London

Wimbledon, and qualified in medicine at St Mary's. He was appointed Professor of Medicine at St Mary's at the remarkably young age of thirty four. His academic output was remarkable. He was a Trustee of the Wellcome Trust from 1975 to 1994 and Deputy Chairman from 1991 to 1994. Following retirement he was appointed Master of the Hunterian Institute of the Royal College of Surgeons from 1988 to 1992. I sat on the Council of the Royal College of Surgeons in my capacity as President of the Royal College of Radiologists when Stan attended. I think he enjoyed this experience as much as I. Stan is a man of great character, a leader in medicine, encouraging when he detects talent and intolerant of mediocrity and apathy. Slim in build, articulate in speech and expressive in presentation, he attracts attention naturally. His days were devoted to his work with a constancy only equalled by his love for Peggy his wife. He is an ardent skier and tennis player and still does both although now past eighty years of age.

Stan and I have had many happy times together. We appeared on stage at the medical school Christmas soirée with a group of consultants that mimed to pop music. The group varied from time to time but participants were, Harold Edwards, neurologist, Dick Wilcox, venereologist, Ian Kenyon, vascular surgeon, Granville Grossman, psychiatrist, Stan Peart, Professor of Medicine, Felix Eastcott, vascular surgeon, Barry Hulme, nephrologist, Peter Richards, physician and later Dean, and myself. We enjoyed the performances but the best fun was the rehearsals, and getting our stage make-up put on by medical student girls. It was rare for consultants to appear on the student stage but Harold Edwards and I thought it a good idea and got the team together. I think the students liked it.

The most medically gifted of my colleagues have been colourful characters and perhaps London teaching hospitals attract such doctors. Other professions no doubt attract similar men and women but my experience lies in medicine. Such characters have their difficulties, as John Webster wrote in *The Duchess of Malfi*, 'physicians are like kings, they brook no contradiction'. It is rare for such characters not to be selfcentred, selfish and at times extremely difficult and argumentative, but I believe the price to pay for their excellence is worth it.

An exceptionally gifted colleague at St Mary's was George Bonney, an orthopaedic surgeon. His life was moulded by his schooling in Eton where he was a scholar. I have known few men so affected by their school or so proud of its eminence. George described the rival Harrow as, 'a boys' school in a north London suburb'. This 'tongue in cheek' remark is typical of the man and his incisive humour. He qualified in medicine at St Mary's and served in the Royal Naval Volunteer Reserve during the war. George is a large man in every way, tall and broad. His major claim to excellence is his international reputation for the repair of damaged brachial plexus nerves (nerves supplying the arms). It's difficult to convey how much this demands the most delicate precision and accuracy. Few can do it. His skill extends to his general orthopaedic work but his reputation soars to Olympian heights in the neurological surgery of the spine and brachial plexus. He is a very temperamental man with a finely honed sense of humour. Widely educated and highly intelligent he is dismissive of those less so and apt to show it. I remember on one occasion he delivered an after-dinner speech at the Royal College of Physicians, entirely in Latin. Few could understand it,

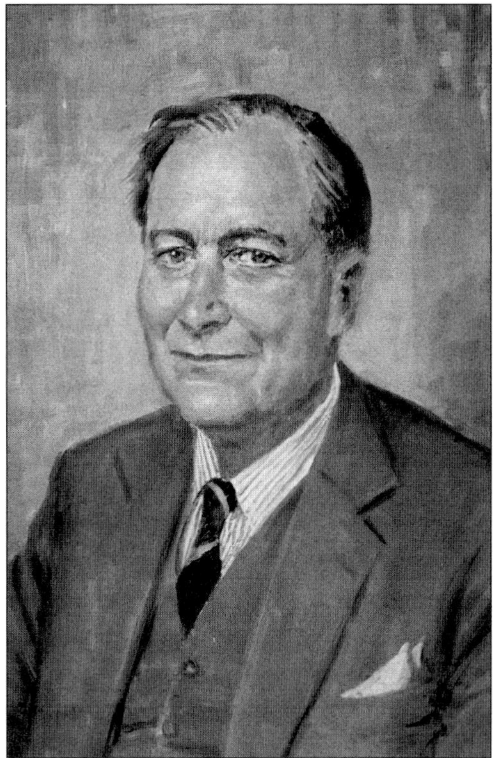

Mr George Bonney FRCS. Consultant Orthopaedic Surgeon, St Mary's Hospital, Paddington, London

but it was delivered with much gesticulation and in such a 'throw-away style' as to be hilarious and was enjoyed by everyone.

George has written extensively and included another of his special interests, in the field of medical negligence. He was an adviser to the Medical Defence Union, which like the Medical Protection Society deals with medical litigation, (I held a similar post with the Medical Protection Society). At one time George chaired the Medical Committee of St Mary's Hospital, but I regret it was a time when the committee was losing its power to administrators.

An indication of George's wide interests is that in retirement he wrote a book, *The Battle of Jutland*, a work of great scholarship. Despite a very busy medical life he has found time to pursue his hobbies of fishing and shooting. Worthy sports for such a man! It's perhaps a cliché to say we do not see men of this character or excellence today, but I have not seen anyone of George's unique quality in the making. He has enriched our lives by knowing him.

An eccentric and gifted senior colleague who died many years ago was Arthur Dickson Wright. Dickson Wright was a brilliant surgeon, perhaps the most capable surgeon in the United Kingdom of his time. He was one of the last, if not the last, of the general surgeons . His operating list was extraordinary so often. He would perform a procedure on the brain, then perhaps another on the chest and proceed to an abdominal case, even pin a fractured hip and finish with the surgery of varicose veins. No surgeon today could or would undertake such a width of procedures in the United Kingdom. Nor would it be recommended. This is the age of fine specialization and indeed the high level of medical litigation would make stepping outside special skills hazardous. Such diverse procedures may still be done by single surgeons in remote areas of the world. There is the story of the medical officer during the Vietnam War in a remote jungle setting called upon to do a surgical procedure of which he had little or no experience. He prayed, 'Lord, in better times, use better men, but now, Lord – use me.' Most medical men would accept the need to try under extreme circumstances and there are surely many who have done so. Dickson Wright was also a gifted speaker and again perhaps the best known medical after dinner speaker of his day. I first heard him lecture when he visited Trinity College, Dublin and I was a very young medical student. I didn't realize I would join the staff of St Mary's so many years later while he was still the senior surgeon. Dickson was cast in the mould of the archetypal surgeon, dictatorial, blunt and self-assured. Many times I've admired the confidence he portrayed. He had a gruff manner, but his authoritarian attitude transferred his confidence to the patient. Invariably this was well placed. He was medium in height, stocky in build, always dressed in black coat, striped trousers and polka dot bow tie. He had a wicked sense of humour and was the greatest gossip I've known in my medical career. Loved by the students for his caustic wit, he was a legend in his own time for his teaching as well as his surgery. His tendency to gossip and his sharp tongue tended to make enemies rather than friends. He was also feared by many. A distressing habit he had in later years was to pick a victim during a speech and to raise a laugh at his expense. The victim of his choice was invariably a professorial colleague. I've told the story frequently that when he had made a diagnosis he would often say to the patient, 'Do you want to be treated academically or do you want to be cured?'

Dickson made his own rules and played fast and loose with the National Health Service. He would turn up late for his clinics if he turned up at all. Fortunately he had a good team who dealt with this. His time keeping for the theatre was equally lax. Today this wouldn't be acceptable. I heard it said he didn't take his Health Service salary. His private practice was so large he didn't need it. His work load was enormous and he worked incessantly well into the night. This put a load onto his team who loyally bore it. To have worked for and with Dickson Wright was the reward.

Dickson had an Irish background, his father was a physician in Dublin. His early surgical career was in Singapore where he was Professor of Surgery. Apart from his consultancy at St Mary's Hospital he had sessions at the Prince of Wales Hospital, Tottenham. He was a Vice-President of the Royal College of Surgeons and a Hunterian Orator. He held the Presidencies of the British Society of Neurological Surgeons, the Medical Society of London, the Hunterian Society and the Harveian Society of London. He raised vast sums of money while the Honorary Treasurer of the Imperial Cancer Research Fund. He listed his hobbies in *Who's Who* as – Nil. Not long after his retirement he had a stroke which removed his two remarkable skills, his manual dexterity and his speech. He languished in the Lindo Wing of St Mary's Hospital for three years. Some weekends I had him to my home for tea but he wasn't happy in this domestic scene. Despite the vast sums he raised for cancer and his surgical excellence he received no honours. This was a pity. I admired Dickson Wright's surgical skill, and I wished I had some of his panache, but since his death he has had bad publicity from his daughter. Clarissa Dickson Wright has declared publically that her father was brutal and that she and her mother were physically abused at home. She states he was a chronic alcoholic. I cannot say what went on in Dickson Wright's home. I know nothing of his physical violence, but believe he could be capable of it. What I do know is that he never appeared in the hospital at any time to be drunk. I attended many hospital and medical school dinners when he was present. He never drank to excess and never appeared drunk on any occasion. Clarissa admits too, she never heard any complaints about his operating.

Harry Hubert Grayson Eastcott, always known as Felix, was a consultant vascular surgeon at St Mary's Hospital. Felix, small in build, is a giant in vascular surgery. It was he who brought back from America the skill and the drive to make vascular surgery successful in the United Kingdom. Others were quick to follow his lead and St Mary's became a hospital acknowledged internationally for its work in this field. Felix published extensively and wrote a definitive book, *Arterial Surgery* which was published in 1969 and has had numerous editions since then. He has lectured in major centres worldwide. Following qualification he served in the Royal Naval Volunteer Reserve during the war. He holds numerous Fellowships and was Honorary Surgeon to the Royal Academy of Dramatic Arts. Felix was Vice-President of the Royal College of Surgeons and President of the Medical Society of London. He read my citation when I was awarded the Fellowship of the Royal College of Surgeons ad eundem. He was also one of my sponsors when I joined the Garrick club. Another was Harold Edwards. Felix is a surgeon of skill and distinction. Unlike many surgeons he has a quiet, self-effacing manner. He is a kind compassionate man and a talented pianist. In retirement he still attends clinical meetings and his opinion is still valued although now over eighty years of age. He remains agile and bright as ever.

A colleague nearer to my age was George Pinker, later Sir George, obstetrician and gynaecologist at St Mary's Hospital. George was appointed obstetrician and gynaecologist to Her Majesty Queen Elizabeth from 1973 to 1990. He was President of the Royal College of Obstetricians and Gynaecologists from 1987 to 1990, and following that President of the Royal Society of Medicine. George qualified at St Mary's in 1947. He and I were members of the Conference of Medical Royal Colleges now the Academy, when I was President of the Royal College of Radiologists. We both also had consultancies at the Bolingbroke Hospital in Wandsworth. In fact it was George and another colleague, Eric Nieman, a neurologist, who persuaded me to take sessions there, which I never regretted. George is an archetypal obstetrician, silver haired at an early age, handsome and charming. He was loved by his patients to whom he gave undivided attention and care. He has a strong personality and like many of my colleagues has a determination when fighting for what he wishes for his specialty. Accordingly he speaks his mind clearly and positively. This is an attribute when directed toward hospital, medical school and college affairs. He is popular with his colleagues and with the students. He has always demonstrated a loyalty to St Mary's Hospital and its medical school despite the enormous call on his time throughout the United Kingdom and abroad. Like the colleagues I've mentioned already he is retired now and like them his interest in the affairs of the hospital and medical school remains as strong as ever.

While George was a medical student he appeared in the medical school productions of Gilbert and Sullivan. I never saw him perform, not having been at St Mary's at the time, but many have told me what a superb voice he had. This led to invitations to join the D'Oily Carte Opera Company. He didn't, but I wonder if he was tempted. A memorable performance of *The Mikado*, in which he starred, was held in the medical school, attended by the Duke and Duchess of York, Elizabeth and Margaret (later the King and Queen, Queen Elizabeth and Princess Margaret). Little did he know he would in mature years become the Royal obstetrician and gynaecologist. George looked after my daughter Louise for the birth of my first grandson, William. He lists his hobbies in *Who's Who* as music, gardening, sailing, skiing and fell walking. I'm surprised he found time for them!

A colleague who I see quite often in retirement is John Crawford Adams, consultant orthopaedic surgeon to St Mary's Hospital. John is eighty seven years old this year and still active in mind and body. He qualified in medicine in 1937 and was a specialist in the Royal Air Force Volunteer Reserve during the war. Later he became the Civilian Consultant in Orthopaedic Surgery to the Royal Air Force. I saw much of John during his consultancy at St Mary's. I admired his surgical skill, but especially his unique approach to orthopaedic problems. Primarily John is a thoughtful, conservative physician, not common in my experience in orthopaedic surgeons. When we were both in practice, John consulted me often to discuss the diagnosis in difficult and rare orthopaedic problems. I often wondered if he needed to as he invariably had the diagnosis. We developed a rapport which also is not common between radiologists and orthopaedic surgeons. John has always been a prodigious writer even in retirement. His book *Outline of Orthopaedics*, first published in 1956, is in its 12th edition and is acknowledged as a definitive text internationally. His *Outline of Fractures* had its 10th edition published in 1992. He has written many other books and

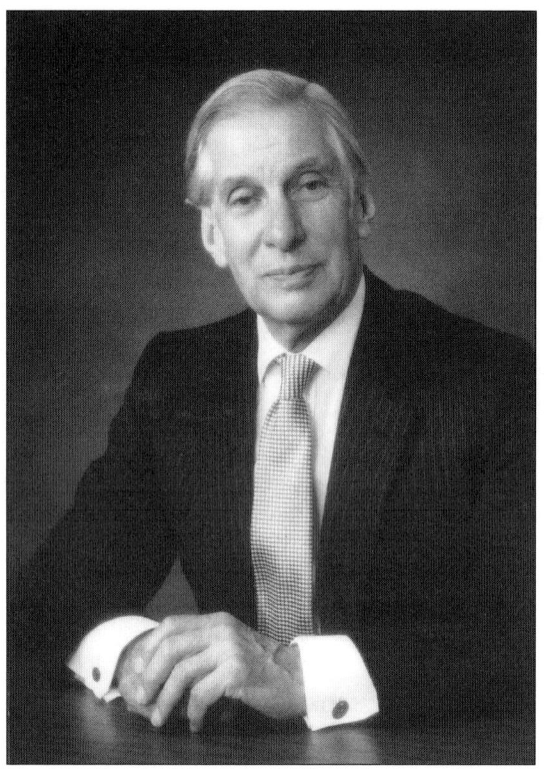

Mr John Crawford Adams FRCS. Consultant Orthopaedic Surgeon, St Mary's Hospital, Paddington, London

chapters in books. He was Production Editor of the *Journal of Bone and Joint Surgery*. In retirement John wrote *Shakespeare's Physic, Lore and Love*. This is an unique account of the medical conditions mentioned in Shakespeare's works. John also finds time to pursue his hobby as a silversmith and his home is graced by many examples of his skill. Some years ago, a cousin, John Dowey, living in Northern Ireland, asked me to recommend an orthopaedic surgeon in London to operate on his hip. 'John, I think the best man to do your particular operation is John Crawford Adams. He is extremely skilled and is a leader in his field.'

'Where does he work?'

'At St Mary's Hospital.'

'I'll think about that and phone you again.' Some weeks later he telephoned.

'Oscar, about the operation, I think that surely the best surgeons for hip operations must be in the Royal National Orthopaedic Hospital.'

'Yes, they are excellent, but I would recommend John Crawford Adams.'

'I think I'll go to the Orthopaedic Hospital.'

'Well John, you must do what you think best.'

John Dowey was successfully operated upon at the Royal National Orthopaedic Hospital. After the operation he spoke to the surgeon. 'Could you tell me exactly what you did at the operation?'

'Well, Mr Dowey, I did a John Crawford Adams procedure.' He explained this. John Dowey to his credit, laughed as he told me this, but my laughter was louder.

An extraordinary man is Professor Hugh Dudley, CBE, Professor at St Mary's Hospital Medical School from 1973 to 1988. Hugh came to St Mary's at a time when the surgical unit needed a strong leader. This they got. Educated in Heath Grammar School, Halifax, Edinburgh and Harvard Universities he qualified in Edinburgh in 1947 winning the Gold Medal and Chiene Medal. He is a Fellow of the Surgical Colleges of England, Edinburgh and America and was a Research Fellow in Harvard University. Before coming to St Mary's he held the post of Foundation Professor of Surgery, Monash University, Melbourne, Australia. Hugh has an incisive and original mind. He leads and stimulates research in surgery and has published extensively, his books running into many editions. His skills as an author extend to many non-medical topics. He was Chairman of the Editorial Board of the *British Journal of Surgery*, Associate Editor of the *British Medical Journal* and Chairman of the Medical Writers Group. He guided the surgical unit at St Mary's conscientiously, working incessantly. Hugh has a quick temper, feared by many, and doesn't take kindly to woolly thinking. This was often seen at the weekly clinical staff rounds attended by the hospital consultants, their teams and students. It was also displayed on occasions at committee meetings in the hospital and medical school. Beneath this at times forbidding temperament, lay a caring, conscientious man, dedicated to surgery. He was also driven by a strong sense of intellectual honesty. There are few men who don't seek praise or favour but Hugh is one. In *Who's Who* he lists one of his hobbies as 'annoying people'. For St Mary's he was a man of substance, a motivator and a colleague I admired. He retired to Scotland and I regret I don't see more of him.

Hugh and I shared a friend in Lance Bromley, a consultant chest surgeon at St Mary's. Lance was one of my referees when I applied for a consultant post at St Mary's. I wrote my first major clinical paper with Lance Bromley and my then chief Rohan Williams on lung changes during surgery. The cases researched were patients operated upon by Lance. I was appointed Visiting Consultant to Gibraltar and made my first trip with Lance who had a similar appointment in surgery. We shared happy times.

Lance attended St Paul's school in London and did his preclinical studies in Caius College, Cambridge. His clinical studies were at St Mary's Hospital Medical School. When he was appointed consultant at St Mary's his surgical load was heavy, as he was the only cardiothoracic surgeon on the staff. He was in fact always on call for his patients. This was to last for many years. His surgery was impeccable and his scrupulous sense of duty to his work was an example for all. When he retired he spent some years as Director of Medical and Health Services in Gibraltar.

Lance is a quiet, gentle, modest man, strong willed when necessary, but conscious of others' feelings. He is never one to bully when in authority. His major hobby is sailing and he has had many fulfilling hours in the seas off Gibraltar.

Most of these colleagues were older than me, but there were many of similar age. Roger Bannister, later Sir Roger, was appointed as a consultant neurologist to St Mary's later than my consultancy and is two years younger than me. Roger's achievements are so many that it is difficult to contain them all in a book such as this. He attended the City of Bath Boy's School, University College School, London and proceeded to Exeter and Merton Colleges Oxford. His clinical undergraduate years were at St Mary's Hospital Medical School. He received many prizes, especially in physiology in which he obtained a Mastership in 1952. Roger gained a William Hyde award for research and at a relatively early age demonstrated his remarkably agile and enquiring mind. He matured into one of the most astute and perceptive thinkers I've known in medicine. He has written extensively, served as a junior medical specialist in the Royal Army Medical Corps, chaired innumerable committees including the Sports Council and lectured throughout the United Kingdom and abroad. He was made a Commander of the British Empire, (CBE), in 1955 and Knighted in 1975. He has been honoured by numerous doctorates. Roger is well known world wide for being the first athlete to break the four minute

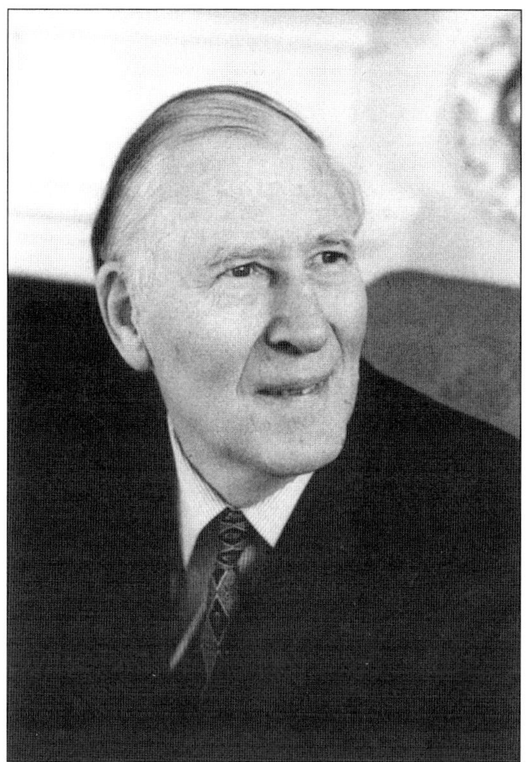

Sir Roger Bannister. Consultant Neurologist St Mary's Hospital, Paddington, London

mile and this was a pivotal achievement of gigantic proportions. Apart from the physical feat, it demonstrated single-minded determination, courage and the mental capacity to push one's resources to the limit of endurance. Roger's consultancies were both at St Mary's and the National Hospital for Nervous Diseases, Queens Square, London. In 1985 he was appointed Master of Pembroke College, Oxford, an appointment worthy of his academic achievements.

A younger colleague was Geoffrey Glazer, consultant surgeon. When I had an attack of acute gall bladder disease, Stan Peart asked me who I wanted to do the surgery. I had no hesitation in saying, Geoffrey Glazer. Geoff qualified at St Mary's in 1964. His surgical reputation is impeccable. He has published widely and produced pivotal papers on disease of the pancreas. He is a doctor's surgeon, trusted by his colleagues for his common sense and his prudent surgery. He is a member of the Court of Examiners of the Royal College of Surgeons

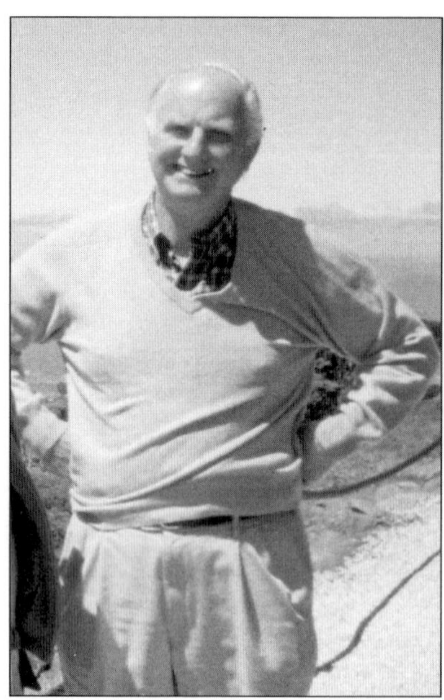

Mr Alasdair Fraser FRCOG. Consultant Obstetrician and Gynaecologist, St Mary's Hospital, Paddington, London

and a Director of Specialist Registrar Training. At a time when medicine and surgery are highly technical Geoff has taught that humanity has not been lost.

A colleague I see quite often in retirement is Alasdair Fraser, obstetrician and gynaecologist. Alasdair qualified at St Mary's in 1955. He is in every sense a St Mary's man and his loyalty to the hospital and medical school is hard to match. Throughout his consultancy at St Mary's he has displayed an enormous interest and concern for the students and their welfare. In addition to teaching them he has supported them in their extra curricula activities, at plays, operas and sporting events. He was President of the St Mary's Hospital Rugby Football Club and recently together with another St Mary's graduate, Frank Horan, wrote a history of the club. I was delighted when Alasdair followed me as Director of Clinical Studies. I thought it a most suitable appointment. Alasdair's interests continued when he was appointed President of the St Mary's Association, for post graduates, and now in retirement his enthusiasm has not slackened. Whenever St Mary's events take place Alasdair will surely be there and remains outspoken for the interests of his alma mater. We dine together often and meet regularly at the Medical Society of London in Lettsom House in Chandos Street.

Perhaps this chapter gives some flavour of St Mary's, but I have only mentioned a few of my colleagues. To mention all would not be possible even though I wished to. Perhaps I will write another book.

Chapter 11

Some Memorable Students

St Mary's hospital had a weakness in the distant past and it was the Casualty Department. It was staffed by junior doctors and there was no senior doctor present on a daily basis. The most able and efficient of the staff was the Casualty sister. Help was available to the junior doctors if they couldn't cope but by and large the situation was unsatisfactory. This changed dramatically with the appointment of a consultant in Accident and Emergency Medicine in 1986. A most remarkable man was appointed, Mr Robin Touquet FRCS. Robin Touquet was educated at Cranleigh School and qualified in medicine at Westminster Hospital Medical School. Having taken some post graduate diplomas he spent some years in general practice. He left general practice to take a large number of surgical posts and obtained his Fellowship of the Royal College of Surgeons in 1979. His academic qualifications were excellent but little was it realized at the time what a strong character this man was and how superb his leadership qualities were. He built up an Accident and Emergency Department of quality entirely due to his drive and determination. The department is the front window of the hospital and as such it shines brilliantly. It was put to a major test recently with the Paddington train disaster and proved its value receiving widespread praise. The department continues to grow and the number of consultants in it has increased. Junior doctors compete to be appointed to work there. The department is acknowledged as an example for others to follow. Robin was a Founding Fellow of the Faculty of Accident and Emergency Medicine and was elected a Faculty Professor in 2002.

He is an example of a graduate from another medical school who has identified totally with St Mary's. Robin has a profound interest in the medical students and follows their progress intently. He is a keen supporter of rugby and was President of the St Mary's Hospital Rugby Football Club from 1994 to 1997 and Joint President of Imperial Medicals Rugby Football Club from 1997 to 2000. His interests with the students also include mountaineering, tennis, athletics and the rifle club.

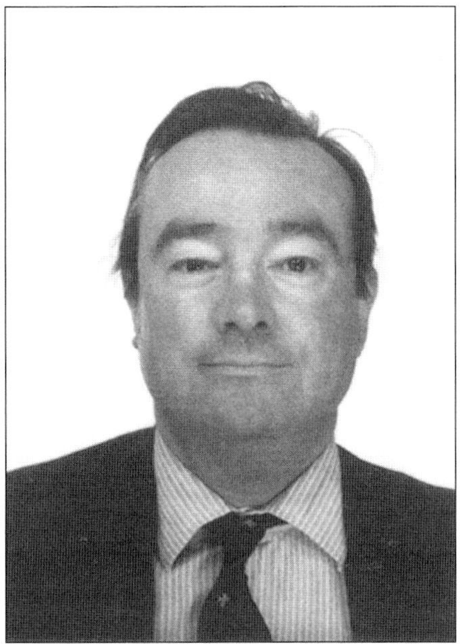

Mr Robin Touquet FRCS. Consultant in Accident and Emergency Department, St Mary's Hospital, Paddington, London

Robin Touquet is an excellent teacher and his strength is also found in the example he gives the students of integrity, loyalty and dedication. He insists on old fashioned values and in his department must be addressed as Mr Touquet at all times by junior staff. His manner is direct and outspoken. Students know exactly where they stand with him and nothing better could be said than that they admire and respect him. So do consultants.

During my medical career I have known a multitudinous number of students. There have been many who were notable characters. It would be impossible to include them all in this text, but I must mention a few.

John Peter Rhys Williams (JPR) was an outstanding rugby player who had fifty five caps for Wales, the first in 1969, and captained the Welsh international side. He took part in innumerable rugby tours and played for the Barbarians. His skill on the rugby field was legendary and indeed he changed the role of the full back. He played for the London Welsh team and for St Mary's in cup matches. His contribution to rugby has been phenomenal. John is a natural ball player and basically an athlete. Few know that he was also a Wimbledon Junior tennis

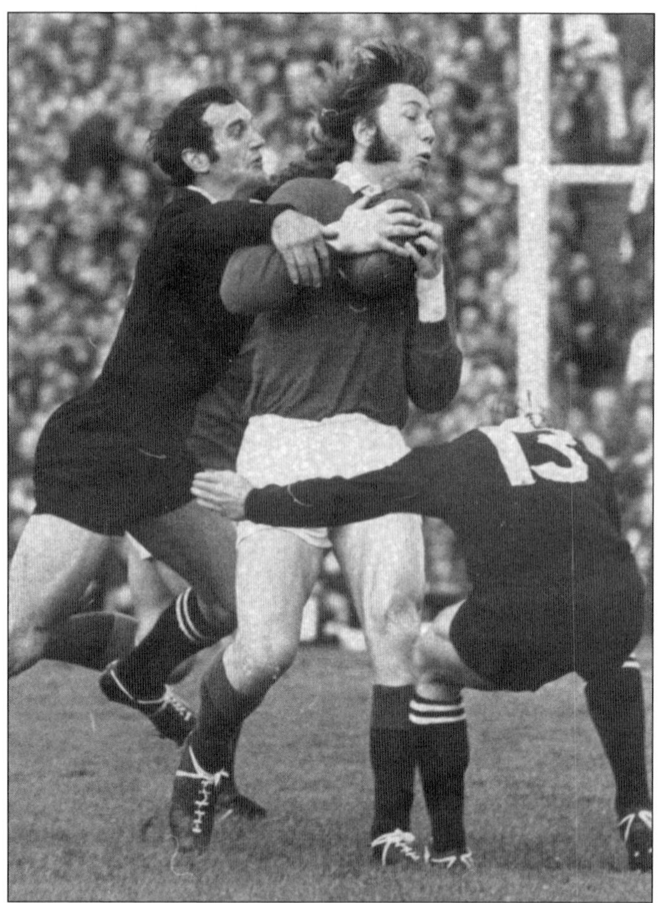

Mr John Williams FRCS (JPR). Consultant Orthopaedic Surgeon. Being tackled by the All Blacks

champion in 1966. John is highly competitive and fearless in the field. This worried me. He had his facial bones broken three times, twice his cheek bone (maxilla) and once his jaw bone (mandible) and suffered innumerable other less dramatic injuries. It was not less dramatic however when he had his face raked by a rugby boot in one highly notorious game.

John took all these injuries in his stride and I wondered if he was impervious to pain.

On the day he had his jaw broken it was wired surgically and he appeared at the official dinner that night. In 1977 he was made a Member of the British Empire (MBE).

I was Director of Clinical Studies when John was a student, and I was concerned that his medical career shouldn't suffer because of his rugby. I had no need to worry, John is intelligent and passed all his examinations. He lost no time because of his rugby and following qualification pursued a career in surgery. He obtained his Fellowship of the Royal College of Surgeons and was appointed a consultant in Trauma and Orthopaedic Surgery at the Prince of Wales Hospital in Bridgend in Wales in 1986.

John is the son of two doctors, the brother of two doctors, Christopher and Philip, the husband of a doctor, Priscilla, (Cilla) and all qualified at St Mary's Hospital. Cilla and John have one son and three daughters, one of whom plays hockey for Wales. Philip, Chris and Cilla are partners in general practice in Bridgend.

The Welsh students who qualified from St Mary's formed the Cambrian Society which holds an annual dinner. I attend as often as possible and am an Honorary member of the Society. I love these dinners where I meet the past students including John, Cilla, Chris and Philip and the evenings are full of good fun and shared memories. Alasdair Fraser also invariably comes.

One of the great strengths of St Mary's is the contribution made to the medical school by the Welsh students. They are an example to all students in the way they take part enthusiastically in the life of the school. They seriously wish to succeed academically but involve themselves in sports, music and drama. They are loyal to the school, courteous and have delightful old fashioned manners. I hope that with the changes in medical education in London we will not lose this Welsh influence. We have need of it.

In November 1984 the BBC began filming a documentary 'Doctors to Be'. They chose ten St Mary's Hospital Medical School students and filmed their progress from the initial interview to qualification and beyond. In the first programme, detailing the interviews, I thought the students came across better than the interviewers. My colleagues often asked questions extremely difficult for young candidates to answer and their assessments of the answers were unreasonably critical. Nonetheless the interview is important and by and large is effective in selecting those most likely to succeed in medicine. The whole series was compulsive viewing, especially for young aspirants wishing to study medicine. The excitement and the trauma of studying medicine were portrayed with reality and the chosen ten spoke and displayed their 'highs and lows' very frankly. Parts of my Freshers Lecture were filmed and repeated in a follow up series. Susan Spindler, television producer and journalist, published an excellent book, *Doctors to Be*, about the series in 1992.

I was disappointed that a proportion of the ten, too high a proportion, were disillusioned with medicine after qualification. I find this difficult to understand but think it's related to the state of the profession in the 1980s and 1990s.

Administrative control in hospital medicine has been largely transferred to non-medical personnel. Since the medical committees have lost administrative control the atmosphere in hospitals has deteriorated. At the moment also there are more lay administrators in the NHS than there are beds. This is a sorry state of affairs. There is also more bureaucracy in general practice.

To save money in the NHS, wards and operating theatres are often closed for long periods and indeed hospitals are closed altogether. Operations are postponed with enormous distress to patients, their families and friends, and to the medical profession.

The working hours of juniors are still too long and fatigue among juniors is commonplace. Patients are more demanding as their expectations are high.

Litigation against the profession was rare when I qualified but now the young doctor is aware that any error, be it significant or not, can lead to a claim in negligence.

The morale in the profession is lower than I have ever known it. These problems do not enter the minds of the student, nor should they, but following qualification they become daily concerns.

One of the ten students in the television series, Fey Probst, was an unusual girl, unaffected by all this during and after qualification. Fey had wished to be a doctor since childhood. She took her A levels at the early age of sixteen and didn't achieve high enough grades to enter medicine. She took the Oxford entrance, succeeded, and read biochemistry. Aged eighteen, she married and left Oxford. She had three children. Fey continued to yearn to read medicine so attended evening classes to improve her A level results. At the time she was pregnant with her fourth child. Aged twenty six she achieved good results and applied for a place at St Mary's. She was granted an interview. Faced with a mature student who at this time was separated from her husband, and had four children to support and care for, the selection panel had a tough decision to make. The selection team on that day was chaired by the Dean, Peter Richards, who says he was prepared to take a gamble with this girl. He moved the committee to accept her, which they did. Fey's enthusiasm for medicine was unequalled by anyone I've known. She was starry eyed almost to the point of absurdity, but it was no flash in the pan. This enthusiasm never left her, and at no stage despite innumerable hardships was she ever disillusioned. I think her home life must have been chaotic and the children had to be to a large degree self sufficient. She attended all lectures, tutorials, ward rounds, outpatients and operating sessions conscientiously, went home, cooked and washed.

The children put to bed she studied until the early hours of the morning. The course was five years and she qualified on time and with high spirits did her pre-registration year's house jobs in medicine and surgery. One of her medical posts was on the Dean's team. While going off duty one night she passed the casualty department and saw a large number of casualties had been brought in. She volunteered to help and stayed working in the department until the early hours of the morning, unknown to the Dean. Nothing could interfere with Fey's fervour. It was realized by the Dean and many colleagues that she would have to control her best instincts at times and pace herself for survival. Survive she did and she obtained her Membership of the Royal College of Physicians. Today she is a consultant in the Accident and Emergency department of Charing Cross Hospital. Knowing her I think this is a suitable post for her talents. Fey is an example of fanatical dedication to medicine, incredible stamina and determination, and I haven't seen her when she wasn't smiling.

Another student I shall never forget is Alain Robert Mitchell Townsend. Alain came to see me before beginning the clinical part of his course, when I was Director of Clinical Studies.

'Dr. Craig, I'd like to take a year off.'

'Really Alain, why do you want to do that?'

'I'd like to read English literature for a year.'

This was met by a long pause while I tried to think how to give him the decision I had already made, without much thought.

'Alain, why do you want to read English literature?'

'Well, medicine is very specialized and there isn't time to read outside the subject. Doctors have a poor general education and I would like to read and widen my horizons.'

'Alain, you are just about to start your clinical studies.'

'Yes, I know that, but I could start that next year.'

'Don't you want to continue in medicine or are you having doubts?'

'I've no doubts whatever, but I think it would be great to improve my education and the extra time would give me an opportunity to meditate'.

He was calm, smiling, self-assured, convincing and charming. I was the one with the doubts.

'Alain, it is my experience that students who take time off from their clinical work to do something so very different often don't come back.'

'I'll come back alright.'

'I don't like the idea. May I suggest that you qualify. If you want to read English literature do so then, but not now.'

I didn't give my approval and at the time I was sure I'd made the right decision.

I'm not so sure now, and in the light of what subsequently happened I think I made the wrong decision.

Alain went on to qualify in 1977. In 1979, just two years later, he obtained his Membership of the Royal College of Physicians. He next achieved a Ph.D. He is Professor of Molecular Biology in Oxford University and for his original research was elected a Fellow of the Royal Society (FRS) in 1992; a remarkable achievement at so young an age. He was a Fellow of Linacre College 1985 to 1998 and is a Fellow of New College Oxford since 1998. Alain also leads and plays in a jazz band. He married Erin Bannister, daughter of Roger Bannister, and has five children. Alain is without doubt one of the most successful of our students and one of the best brains to have graced St Mary's as a student. Alain would have succeeded whatever. I should have let him have his year reading English literature.

Recently I met Alain at Henley Regatta. He greeted me enthusiastically. I felt compelled to say, 'Alain, I should have let you have that year off to read English literature.'

'I too have thought about that. I think you gave the right advice.'

He has lost none of his charm.

Andrew Wakefield qualified from St Mary's Hospital Medical School in 1981. He is the son of an old St Mary's student, now a consultant neurologist in Bath.

Andrew was in some respects a typical St Mary's student. He played rugby for the first XV, was popular with his peers and took part in the school's extracurricular activities. He was a member of the Summer Ball Committee when I was President of the Ball. Andy is a handsome man, with a quiet pleasing manner, hiding a strong will and a determined personality. He married Carmel O'Donovan, a pretty student who specialized in medico-legal medicine. Andy obtained his Fellowship of the Royal College of Surgeons in 1985. Following many surgical posts he obtained an appointment as Wellcome Research Fellow at the Royal Free School of Medicine, and proceeded to Senior Lecturer in Experimental Gastroenterology in the Departments of Medicine and Histopathology. He followed this as Reader and Honorary Consultant and eventually Director of Research and Chairman, Inflammatory Bowel Disease Group.

Andy has numerous scholarships and awards and has written and contributed to over one hundred and twenty scientific papers. He obtained his Fellowship of the Royal College of Pathologists in 2001.

Andrew Wakefield came into the public arena when he reported that he believed the triple MMR (Measles, Mumps and Rubella) vaccine was linked to the development of autism and bowel disease. This was in 1998 and caused considerable anxiety among parents of young children. The arguments regarding his belief rocked the medical establishment. His theory has been denounced by many experts, including Sir Peter Lachmann, an eminent immunologist, but significantly by the Chief Medical Officer and the Department of Health. An investigation by Melanie Philips for the *Daily Mail* reported 'the British and international medical authorities united to dismiss it, scorning his research as worthless and insisting the vaccination was perfectly safe.' However there is strong anecdotal evidence provided by many parents that their children were normal before receiving the triple vaccine. Melanie Philips continued 'he has been mocked, denounced and driven from his job.' Andy visits the United States of America where his theory has some support and at present is continuing his research hoping to provide evidence that will prove he was right all along. He is not without medical support in the United Kingdom, but the medical forces against him are powerful.

I am unable to say whether Andy Wakefield's theory is right or wrong. I include him in this chapter as I admire his courage and his convictions. It is not easy to defy convention and to maintain your opinions in the face of such powerful opposition, but his conviction is sincere and strong. He has been prepared to sacrifice his professional security for these beliefs.

I think of Alec Bourne, another St Mary's man, who sacrificed his professional career when he aborted a young girl raped by soldiers in the early part of the twentieth century, and standing against the law at the time – changed it.

Chapter 12

The Merging of the London Medical Schools

I'M UNAWARE WHO INITIALLY thought that twelve medical schools in London was excessive. Some critics outside London might think so. Lord Flowers, a scientist, Vice Chancellor of the University of London from 1985 to 1990, chaired the University's Working Party on the future of medical and dental resources in 1979–1980. The Flower's Report recommended that the number of medical schools in London should be reduced. Some questions need to be addressed regarding this. Was the aim to reduce the costs of the National Health Service and especially the University costs?. The close working relationship between the NHS hospitals and the medical schools creates funding which in many areas overlaps. Is it necessary to have twelve professorial units in each specialty in London? These units have large staffs and are expensive. There are a multitude of professorial units in each medical school. Would a reduction of medical schools guard against overlapping research projects? Could the money saved be used to better advantage within the university and perhaps within the NHS? There is a shortage of doctors in the United Kingdom: could the number of medical schools be reduced without reducing the number of medical students in training?

I'm sure the discussions on these lines were far reaching and detailed. I don't know the answers. Another problem was that the referral system of patients had changed. Many of the teaching hospitals in London relied on tertiary referrals from hospitals far and wide, to units of special expertise. Since World War Two, the expertise in hospitals throughout the United Kingdom had improved enormously and the need for tertiary referrals decreased considerably. Teaching hospitals in London had to rely on patients coming from their own catchment area. If there wasn't a large residential population in that area, the number of patients referred would decrease. This was a potent reason for St George's hospital in Hyde Park Corner to move to Tooting. This decision proved to be prophetic and wise. St Bartholomew's and the Middlesex hospitals were in areas of low residential population, as were Guy's and St Thomas's hospitals. King's had a large catchment area, as had St Mary's and the Royal London. The Royal Free had moved to Hampstead where there was a large residential population. Teaching hospitals for some time had been finding it necessary to send students to outlying hospitals for part of their training, to make sure they were taught on a sufficiently wide spectrum of patients, even those with a good catchment area. The threat that some medical schools might even close was a real one and a depressing cloud of uncertainty affected every medical school in London for many years.

At an early stage some medical schools appointed a joint Professor in one or two disciplines, but discussions began between medical schools as to pairing which would reduce the number to six. This led to many rumours, much speculation and more uncertainty. There wasn't one medical school in London that wished to lose its identity. St Bartholomew's, the oldest hospital and medical school in London, was especially worried and the men and women of the commercial life of the City of London were aghast at the threat to what they considered their hospital and medical school. Stickers appeared on cars and elsewhere in London – 'Save Barts'.

The feelings were as strong at St Mary's and no doubt other medical schools. Deans of the medical schools faced uncertain years with difficult decisions to make. The vast majority of consultant staff of teaching hospitals in London didn't wish to see the number of medical schools reduced. More questions were necessary. What would happen to the strong sense of identity that was part of each medical school? Would the loss of identity affect the recruitment of students who wished to go to a particular school? What effect would the reduction of medical schools have on the number of doctors trained? If the number of medical students remained the same then the classes would be enormous. If the classes were enormous then there were insufficient teachers for tutorial groups of a manageable size. It seemed likely the tutorial groups would be enormous, thus destroying their purpose. What effect would the reduction of medical schools have on the social life of the students? What would happen to grants to clubs within the existing schools and what effect would any change have on sporting activities? What would happen to scholarships given to individual medical schools which would no longer exist? What would happen to research sponsored by commercial organizations for a particular school?

For a time it was thought that St Mary's would pair with the Middlesex. At the time the consultant staff were against this. Of course they were against any form of pairing, but unable to stop the tide of change.

Peter Richards, the Dean of St Mary's Medical School at the time, began negotiations for St Mary's Hospital Medical School to become part of Imperial College of Science and Technology. This plan, to preserve the medical school without being paired with another, seemed wise at the time, but in the end it led to the loss of St Mary's Hospital Medical School and the birth of Imperial College of Science, Technology and Medicine. The transition isn't easy but is progressing. In the early stages St Mary's students found themselves competing for society and club grants, but Imperial was much larger and more powerful. Even the *St Mary's Medical School Gazette* had to go, and the legendary St Mary's Hospital Rugby Football Club became Imperial Medicals Rugby Club. Great efforts were made to keep a separate medical school choir and orchestra but the identity with St Mary's was lost.

It was to get worse when Charing Cross Medical School and the Westminster Medical School became part of Imperial College and also lost their identity. This merging of medical schools proceeded throughout London. The medical schools have been reduced to five. They are, Kings, Guy's and St Thomas's; St Bartholomew's and the Royal London; University College, the Middlesex and the Royal Free; St Mary's, Charing Cross and the Westminster; and on its own St George's.

For many years I gave the Fresher's Lecture at St Mary's. I lectured to approximately eighty to one hundred students. The number at Charing Cross and the Westminster would have been the same. All these Freshers are now at Imperial and I lecture to over 300 students. This is too large for one lecture theatre and the lecture has to be transmitted to a second theatre, losing some of its impact.

The medical school has moved to a site in Kensington on the Imperial campus. This is miles away from any of the hospitals. There has been a loss of identity with the hospitals and the students spend hours and pounds sterling travelling around London. The rapport of the students with the hospital staff has deteriorated.

The opposition of consultants and medical school staff to the merging of medical schools is mainly because they can see no advantages in doing so apart from finance. There has been no noticeable opposition to these mergers from the Royal Colleges or from the British Medical Association. This is sad. I find it hard to believe that they approve of the changes, and perhaps they stand back thinking it is a decision made by the University of London and are unwilling to interfere. Who knows?

I have been very fortunate in my medical career. I went to St Mary's as a registrar in 1957 and was appointed a consultant in 1963. I retired in 1992 and my years at the hospital and medical school couldn't have been happier. I think St Mary's is special, but I'm aware that consultants in other London teaching hospitals may think the same of their hospital and medical school. Rivalries and feuds between consultants in different disciplines, and sometimes in the same discipline, exist in any hospital but there was no serious friction at St Mary's during my time. There were differences among colleagues, and I also suffered from that, but there was no significant discord. The atmosphere day by day was good. By and large the consultants respected each other. The history of the hospital was such as to generate pride and the number of FRS awards, civic honours and two Nobel prizes for medicine justified this. I developed an unusually strong allegiance to St Mary's which has grown over the years. I loved my association with the students and the postgraduates and my time as Director of Clinical Studies. A great advantage to the spirit of the school was the ratio of staff to students! The consultants and lecturers knew the students well and were interested in their welfare. At a dinner recently a past student, Jackie Seifert (nee Morris), now a consultant physician said, 'The wonderful thing about the students' life at St Mary's was that they received pastoral care individually.'

At the interview of candidates for entry it was the custom to look for students with wide interests as well as academic ability. Extra curricular activities were encouraged and sports excelled as did music and drama. I believe the spirit of St Mary's Hospital Medical School is unique. I believe that the medical school produced doctors of character. There were some disappointments inevitably, but they were few. Many may say I exaggerate or see St Mary's through rosy spectacles, but this is how I feel. I hope the reader will understand my distress therefore when the school joined Imperial and the medical school I loved disappeared. The hospital remains but what is it without the medical school?

This disappointment is shared with my colleagues. It was decided to hold a dinner to mark the demise of the medical school and its union with Imperial. The dinner was titled 'Hail and Farewell'. It was held at the Hurlingham Club and 700 attended. I felt honoured to be asked to give the final speech for the St Mary's Hospital Medical School, even though I had retired some years before. I think it was the speech, of all I've given, that I most wanted to give to pay tribute to the medical school that had adopted me. I reproduce it here, word for word.

Hail and Farewell Dinner
December 1998

Mr Chairman, Ladies and Gentlemen, Colleagues,

When I give my lecture to the Freshers on their first day in the medical school, I say,

'This is the most important day of your life. Nothing will ever be the same again'.

I say to you to-night, This is the most important day of your life. Nothing will ever be the same again it is a pivotal and critical time in the life of St Mary's Hospital Medical School. The union with Imperial has taken place and now we must approach it as a challenge and bring to it all the qualities that make St Mary's special.

However the union does remind me of a story, which certainly applies to our present situation. 'There was a Russian peasant, walking along a country lane in a snowstorm. The weather was atrocious, cold as cold can be. He was huddled into a sheepskin jacket. As he walked along the lane he saw a little bird lying on the ground. It seemed dead, but he picked it up and held it in his hands. He cradled it under his coat and to his surprise he felt a little movement. My God, he thought, it's alive. It moved just a fraction more. At that moment a herd of cattle came into the lane and as they walked toward him they deposited their excreta on the road. The steam rose from the excreta and our peasant had a bright idea. He put the bird into the middle of one of the lumps of excreta from which the steam was rising. The little bird felt the warmth and began to move quite a lot. Soon it wiggled its wings and then began to sing. It whistled and whistled, full of joy. At that moment a fox came along behind the hedge and heard the bird singing. It jumped over the hedge and gobbled up the bird. Eaten, gone.

Now there are three morals to this story.

The man who puts you in the shit, isn't necessarily your enemy.
The man who takes you out of the shit, isn't necessarily your friend.
And when you're in the shit – don't sing about it.'

St Mary's Hospital Medical School was founded by Samuel Lane in 1854, 144 years ago. What a privilege it's been to be part of it. I will recall for you some of the people that have worked in the hospital and medical school. Augustus Desirée Waller who discovered the electrical pathways of the heart and gave us the electrocardiogram. He paved the way for modern cardiology and cardiac surgery. Almroth Wright, the son of a Northern Irish Presbyterian minister, worked at St Mary's for 45 years. He evolved the anti-typhoid vaccine. He was the father of therapeutic immunization and brought medicine into a new era, saving millions of lives. Alexander Fleming discovered penicillin, a dour Scot who again changed the face of medicine and catapulted the medical profession into the antibiotic age where infections previously fatal could be fought and cured. These discoveries alone were world shattering, and earned St Mary's a prime place in history.

Sir Bernard Spilsbury was a renowned forensic pathologist, perhaps the most renowned ever in that specialty. His name was known by every adult in the United Kingdom for his evidence as an expert witness in many famous murder trials. He established the expert witness as a force in the courts. Alec Bourne, obstetrician and gynaecologist, a man of immense moral courage, risked his freedom and his professional life, defying the law at the time, performing an abortion on a 14-year-old girl, the victim of rape. He believed that a doctor must act for what he thinks is in the best interests of the patient, no matter what the cost. He changed the attitude of the people of this country to abortion, leading many years later to changes in the law. I can go on, Barcroft, Price James, Colebrook, Harris, Kettle, all with FRS awards.

In fact we've had over 30 Fellows of the Royal Society at St Mary's. I believe this is more than any other medical school in London. We had the great Dean, Lord Moran, also President of the Royal College of Physicians, and physician to Winston Churchill. Lord Porrit was a Rhodes Scholar, an Olympic athlete, a President of the Royal College of Surgeons, President of the British Medical Association and President of the Association of Surgeons of Great Britain and Ireland, a Queen's surgeon who became Governor of New Zealand. We have had many Presidents of Royal Colleges, the Royal College of Surgeons, Royal College of Physicians, and the Royal College of Obstetricians and Gynaecologists, who recently have been George Pinker and Stanley Simmonds. We have had three Presidents of the Royal College of

Radiologists, Rohan Williams, Rhys Davies and myself. In recent years Felix Eastcott brought vascular surgery to St Mary's and the United Kingdom. He and Ian Kenyon developed vascular surgery to its present excellence. This excellence is continued by Averil Mansfield. Stan Peart discovered the association between hypertension and renal disease, another FRS and a knighthood. Bob Williamson did his pivotal work on the gene of cystic fibrosis. We had two Nobel prizes, Fleming and Porter.

St Mary's has an academic record second to none. This is a unique medical school. You are a special people.

We can boast of winning the Hospital Rugby cup more than any other London medical school, passing Guy's some years ago. We have many caps for England, Wales and Ireland and four captains of England and one captain of Wales. We have excelled in other sports including water polo, hockey, fencing, sailing and mountaineering. We had Olympic oarsmen and fencers and Bannister broke the four minute mile. This is a unique medical school. You are a special people. We have a thriving Dramatic Society, a successful Music Society and a wonderful Symphony Orchestra. This is a unique medical school. You are a special people.

There is indeed a special St Mary's man, a special St Mary's woman, recognizable from the first day of coming to this place. There is a special St Mary's spirit – a strength of character grafted on to St Mary's medical men and women. I will give you two examples.

Ivan Jacklin, a young graduate naval surgeon was on a boat torpedoed in tropical waters during World War Two. The raft on which he lay was overcrowded and a weaker colleague was hanging on to the side. Jacklin said, 'Take my place'. He slipped off the raft and hung on himself. He was taken by sharks during the night.

McCrea was sunk in Artic waters. His raft held 17. There were 18 on it. It was in danger of capsizing. He said, 'I think I'm in the way'. He dived overboard and was never seen again.

This St Mary's spirit lives on.

Our union with Imperial is a fact, but I want to say to you in the words of Dylan Thomas,

'Do not go gentle into that good night,
Rage, rage against the dying of the light.'

We want the spirit of St Mary's to go to this Imperial union and last for a thousand years so that in the words of Churchill, people will say – 'This was their finest hour.' The spirit of St Mary's must never die.

Chapter 13

Holidays

Since writing the last chapter Nancy and I have been for a weekend to Wissant, a small fishing village about 20 kilometres south of Calais. For many years we holidayed in France, mainly in Brittany. When we had only two children and there were 11 francs to the pound we stayed in modest hotels. When we had four children, a large mortgage and there were less francs to the pound (I remember when it was seven), we tried camping. We hired a continental tent. I had never erected a continental tent and I'm not good at such things. I even find the instructions difficult to follow. I decided to erect it in the garden before leaving to make sure I could do it when we arrived at the camp site in France. This first attempt proved a great source of amusement to my four young girls and supported by their mocking mother, they made my task more difficult. I ended up in a mess with the tent flaps inside instead of outside and one side of the tent unsupported and flapping. There also appeared to be too few long supporting rods but yet I had some small rods with nowhere to put them. My family was laughing hilariously.

'You won't find this so funny when we're in camp in France and you wish to have a meal or go to bed.'

Nancy then looked at the instructions and together with the children we all managed to get it right. I'm not a DIY man at all. I'm so glad we practised before we left.

One night in the camp as I prepared for bed I had to call Nancy.

'Darling, there's a large frog sitting on my pillow.'

Nancy replied with a smile,

'I'm sure there's room for both of you.'

'Very funny, but I want you to get rid of it.'

'How do you suggest I do that?'

'I don't know. Put it in a bucket.'

I got one of the girls' beach buckets and gave it to her.

I turned my back and bravely didn't watch.

'It's gone.'

A few night's later there was a thunderstorm and the lightening was fierce and frightening as the torrential rain drummed on the canvas. Nancy woke up and said, 'That's a bad storm.'

'Yes, and what's worse we're under trees and that's dangerous.'

Nancy sat up.

'Why did you tell me that.'

'Well, it's true.'

'You're trying to frighten me.'

'No, I'm not, but in any case I can't sleep on this hard lino bed with that drumming sound. You seem to be quite comfortable.'

'I was until you mentioned the trees. Should we move?'

'In this storm? Go back to sleep.'

We tried camping only once.

For our next holiday we tried pulling a caravan. I thought this would be much more comfortable than lying in a tent. Full of excitement we went to Gomshall in Surrey to view caravans for hire. Nancy and the girls went into one after another amid shouts of appreciation of their layout and decor. In each the girls picked their beds, unfolded those that required it and lay on each. Dividing doors were tested and the loo in each inspected. Tables were erected and stowed and for reasons I'll never understand, curtains closed and opened. Questions were asked about awnings. I feared I was going to be into another assembly job. When they thought the caravans were too small I knew I should have gone on my own. The owner of the site said, 'Ah yes, I've a larger one in the next shed.'

It was big. Mother and daughters went into overdrive and again tested every table, bed, and window and especially loved the cooking facilities.

'Father, its got a fridge.'

Without consulting me they chorused,

'This is the one we like. We'll take it.'

I was worried. 'I don't think my car is large enough to pull this one.'

The proprietor looked at me,

'What car do you have?'

'An Austin Cambridge Estate.'

'Oh, that's alright. It'll easily handle this.'

I recognized defeat.

I'd never pulled a caravan and here I was with this enormous one. When on the road I realized I couldn't reverse with it on. When this daunting thought struck me I stopped the car and sat with my head in my hands.

Nancy said, 'What's the matter?'

'I can't reverse.'

'Well, do you need to?'

'We'll need to at some time.'

'Why worry about it now?'

'It'll be too late to worry when I have to reverse.'

I tried to go back. The caravan went in the opposite direction, and I couldn't work out the correct manoeuvre to straighten up. As I tried to manipulate the steering, things got worse and the caravan formed a large V with the car. I was looking into one of the windows of the caravan on my right.

Nancy turned her full gaze on me, 'Why can other people reverse with a caravan?'

'I don't know. If I knew that, I'd be able to do it.'

'Can't you try?'

'That's what I'm doing.'

'You're not being very successful, are you?'

The girls remained quiet and I knew things were desperate.

Nancy continued,

'Straighten the car and start again.'

I didn't know if I could straighten the car and the caravan at the same time. I put my head in my hands again.

'What are you doing now?'

'I'm thinking.'

It may not have been the right solution, but it was the only one I could manage. I got out of the car and unhitched the caravan. With help from my critics and a great deal of shouting, I moved the caravan back, adjusted the car and then hitched the caravan on again. This was a major exercise and one I knew couldn't be done on a major road. If I was to get anywhere it was essential I shouldn't pass a road I should have taken. Navigation would be the serious job. I would have my hands full driving, so Nancy must do the navigation. Ha, Ha, Ha!

As we approached Paris I told Nancy, 'We must go around Paris and not through it. It's against the law to pull a caravan through the centre of Paris in the rush hour.'

Someone told me that. I don't know whether it's true or not but it should be.

'Now look carefully at the map and direct me to the peripherique which will go around the city.'

I don't know how we found ourselves driving up the Champs Elysées towards the Arc de Triomphe, with cars hooting all around me, occupants gesticulating and making hideous faces. It was a nightmare.

I found out if you change direction quickly or even if the wind blows the sway of the caravan transmits itself to the car which wobbles and tilts to the point of overturning.

This is especially serious if the car is too light for the size of the caravan. Why had he said my car was right for this caravan? As we swayed dangerously, I heard shrieks of terror from the mother and four daughters. We slowed up and endured further hooting from behind and gesticulating when they passed. I carried on regardless until we were past danger and on a safe and quiet road outside Paris where I stopped. My nerves were shattered. It was time for a break and time to recover.

Nancy decided to cook lunch. Soon eggs were frying in a pan, sizzling in the fat. I couldn't believe it, but a passing lorry was so close that the caravan shook and the lunch, eggs, fat and pan landed on the floor. There were more shrieks from my daughters and their mother. I said nothing but thought I'd never expose myself to this again. We only caravanned once.

When I travelled to lecture or attend meetings in Manchester. Leeds or elsewhere beyond Watford, I went by train. For part of the journey the train ran parallel to the canal north of London. I saw narrow boats glide along, the occupants relaxed and obviously enjoying a peace I longed for in my busy life. It all looked so romantic.

There were boats of every size, each decorated in their own particular style of Barge Art. I admired the painted hulls, green or black with bright red edging, colourful painted flowers and lace covered windows (are they portholes?). If only I owned one of them, but hold on, how often could I use it? However the more I saw the more I longed. It was then I decided to hire one for a holiday. This was exciting but daunting. Surprisingly, it was easy to persuade Nancy and the girls. Louise wished to bring a friend, Roger, and Siobhan invited her boyfriend Chris. So with Finella, Sheena, Nancy and I, we were eight. I needed a big boat.

We hired a very long narrow boat in Iver and I planned to take it as far up the Grand Union Canal and back as I could in a week. The choice of canal was the first mistake. There are thirty six locks between Iver and Aylesbury, and there and back means seventy two locks in a week. They were hand operated locks at the time and may still be so. I've never steered a boat, so I listened carefully to the instructions about starting, stopping, tying up, permitted speeds and rules for the working of the locks. What they didn't tell me was that it takes an inordinately long time between starting to manoeuvre the boat and the boat executing the manoeuvre. To change direction you have to commence the operation long beforehand. When you enter a lock, it's too late to slow the forward movement. You must cut your engine some way before the lock and put the engine in reverse just on entering. It takes some experience to know when to cut the engine as you approach. If you apply the reverse too late this heavy boat will do considerable damage to itself, the lock and any other boat that is already there. With all on board I demonstrated entering locks and explained the manoeuvre to everyone, once I'd become familiar with the technique.

Chris was eager to show his manliness and skill to Siobhan and indeed to us all and begged to take the helm. Hair-raising entries into locks were the result. Roger who had been in narrow boats before was more reluctant to take control.

My ageing body had difficulty coping with so many locks. Nancy worried I might have a coronary attack. Fortunately the two boys competed to show their strength and skill. Nancy told the girls they mustn't jump onto dry land as the boat rose in the lock, but a photograph seen subsequently showed Sheena, my youngest, doing just that. We were terrified someone would fall in and be crushed between the boat and the lock side. Suprisingly, the only one to fall in was Roger, the most experienced on board, but fortunately it was while walking backwards holding the forward rope on leaving a lock. He was very wet and humbled.

Emptying chemical toilets was no fun, but the week was most memorable for the constant rain, and the dampness in the cabin, in the bunks and in the blankets which persisted for the seven days. I wore new jeans and my white underpants turned a bright blue, each day. Nancy confessed that at one stop, she and Siobhan went to a local shop and on seeing a bus marked London, seriously considered desertion.

One morning owing to a bargee leaving a lock gate open we found ourselves tilted significantly to one side on dry land. The canal was devoid of any water in that stretch. It was a long time before we were afloat again. On the way back following many near misses, Chris said, 'I believe it's best to cut the engine before you reach the lock and then put the engine in reverse on entering the lock.'

Much to my surprise I didn't say a word. That holiday was hard work, not at all peaceful and didn't provide the idyllic image I'd seen from the train. We arrived back, wet and cold, tired and tense.

When we think of it now many years later, we think we enjoyed it in some perverse way and although we only had one holiday on a narrow boat, we again watch passing narrow boats thinking we could try it again. Some sunny days I think – perhaps, but the next day it's – perhaps not.

For many years after that we hired gites. I thought this was the solution and so it proved to be most of the time. We did this for years and as the girls got older the number of friends coming with us grew. My Jaguar was full but the rest came by boat, train or in their own cars. Boyfriends and girlfriends changed often, but it was fun and I loved every holiday we had. The best gite we had was in Montcontour. It was approached along a sand track across a field. As I drove to it I was sure we were lost. There couldn't be a house approached like this. We rounded a corner and *mon Dieu*, there was a large gate opening onto a courtyard in which sat a very large imposing house, almost a small chateau. I thought we were in the wrong place but then saw two cars, one belonging to my eldest daughter Siobhan and her husband Chris, and the other to Robin Bruce, their friend from Ewell in Surrey. What a sight. The grounds were massive and contained two lakes. There were outhouses, with a tractor in one, a source of great pleasure for Siobhan's young son. Ted and Celia Goodacre, our friends from Ewell, were with us and liked the area so much, that they looked for a suitable house to buy. They found one in the village but after much debate decided it was too small, and difficult to get to for weekends.

Robin Bruce loved the place and would take a boat into the middle of one of the lakes with a box of beer and consume the lot. On one occasion we got anxious.

'Where's Robin?'

'He went out in the boat with a load of beer.'

'But he's been gone a long time. Too long.'

'Gosh, yes he has. We'd better look for him.'

We all rushed to the lake. There was the boat in the middle but we couldn't see Robin. We all started to shout at once.

'Robin, Robin, Robin!'

Nothing happened. Shout again.

'Robin, Robin, Robin!'

A face appeared above the boat.

'What's wrong?'

'Nothing. Go back to sleep.'

We had a wonderful holiday and went back the next year. That was many years ago and I'd like to go back again.

Siobhan and Chris live and work in Paris. Some years ago they bought a mobile home near Calais for weekends. Nancy and I often met them for lunch in Calais, travelling on the ferry from Dover as foot passengers. One day they brought us for lunch in Wissant a small fishing village in the Pas de Calais. We ate in the Hotel de Plage. The meal and wine were good. We were amused when the waitress, wearing a short tight black dress, came from the kitchen with the imprint of a large hand on her bottom. It wasn't there when she went in. In the centre of the village we saw the Normandy Hotel and liked it immediately. For the last twelve years Nancy and I stayed there at least twice or thrice a year. The hotel owner, Monsieur Davies, was born in Wissant, with a Welsh father and a French mother. Before World War Two the family owned a garage and a small hotel restaurant. During the war as the German army entered Wissant, the family were leaving on the road to Calais. They were fortunate to get on a boat and went to Wales where they spent the remainder of the war. The rush to get out was such that the youngest son was left behind. This was difficult for them all but especially the one left in Wissant. The present owner of the hotel was a boy of nine at the time and I'm unaware of the age of his younger brother. When the war was over they returned to Wissant and the present hotel came into existence and is improving year by year. The boy of nine is now seventy one years old and in the last few years his son, Didier Davies manages the business. The hotel is basic French, clean and serves good food and wine. It is remarkably inexpensive and Nancy and I find it a wonderful place to relax, enjoy the beaches and eat and drink to a level of pleasure difficult to find this side of the channel. Only once did we have a disappointing evening and it wasn't the fault of the hotel or the French.

There is little to see in this seaside village, a square, a few shops, a post office and a grey stone church. In the morning the fishing boats are pulled up from the beach, sit in the square and oil-skinned fishermen sell the night's catch from the boats, while others untangle the nets with rough hewn hands. Alongside the boulangerie and charcuterie the hotel sits with brown wooden painted beams and cream walls more like Alsace than the Pas de Calais. Tables line the path outside and the sea air is perfumed with coffee and Gauloises. The car park is full with Belgian, Dutch and French cars but few British. There's nothing here for the Brits. They pass it to go south. There's no noise, no fanfares and no amusement arcades. We love to sit and watch the locals strolling by to get their daily bread, so fresh and crisp. There is little haute couture here.

Our room is sparce but has a large bathroom and we need no more. We've been in Hong Kong Mandarins and Pasadena Ritz Carltons many times. Here all is peace.

We pass the time relaxed between each meal. Why is the wine so much better than at home? We drink a full-bodied red and our spirits rise with each mouthful. We drink slowly and deliberately delighting in each moment. Perhaps we don't buy the right wine at home.

One quiet day we swam, bobbing in the warm salt waves. The only sound was the gentle soothing movement of the sea. We changed for dinner and ate at eight. We had plaice with a creamy smooth sauce, a bottle of Sancerre, cool from the ice. Life was tranquil. We'd left the world to settle all its woes. It couldn't reach us here.

After dinner we walked gently to the beach in the humid, calm night. There was a crimson sun, with vibrant streaks of red, a Turner's sky of unsurpassing beauty.

The sea and sand stretched into the night, the silence like a gift from God. We loved it. We turned and took the road back.

And then I saw the woman run towards our path, a boy of five or so clutching her hand. In violent pursuit was a lean shaven headed man, agile and bent in speed, shouting 'Shut your fuckin' mouth, you fuckin' woman.'

She cried, 'Why do you keep hitting me?'

'Shut your fuckin' mouth. Why tell the man? Shut your fuckin' mouth.'

I looked at this Englishman and felt disgust and shame. I couldn't see the face of her poor child and I'm thankful for that as it would haunt me. They ran down another street – and I walked on. The day was dead. That lout had killed it.

That was my only bad experience in twelve years in Wissant.

Some years ago I was talking to my friend Professor Robert Steiner and his wife Gertie about Wissant. They wished to join us on a holiday there, so we planned a few days at the Normandy Hotel. Another friend Dr Diana Brinkley asked to join us. Five fitted into my car and we drove to Dover to take the ferry. It took one and a quarter hours to Dover and the crossing to Calais another one and a quarter hours.

In Calais we took the coast road south, the D940. We drove through Sangatte and then Escalles. The roads were empty and passed rolling fields, large without hedges and stretching for miles beneath a never-ending sky. We passed Cap Blanc Nez and into Wissant, nestling between it and Cap Gris Nez, *la terre de deux caps*. The journey from Calais took only twenty minutes. The cliffs fell down from each Cap to beautiful sandy beaches. The beach at Wissant is sand for seven miles. Nancy and I were anxious lest the hotel would be disappointing as our friends were all seasoned travellers, but our anxiety proved unfounded. They found the hotel adequate and the food more so. We sat the next morning in the square watching the weekly market, sipping coffee as only the French can make it. Robert and I were treated to a young lady trying on hats at a stall. Her back was to us but her legs were exquisite accentuated by her short dress. We laughed about our male preferences and Gertie said, 'If I followed a pair of lovely legs in the Hammersmith Hospital they'd end up in Robert Steiner's office.'

We took a photograph of this girl's legs to give to Robert as a memoir. On subsequent visits on market days we looked for her but we never saw her again.

Some years earlier Siobhan and Chris took us to a restaurant, La Marie Galante, in Audresseles, just a few miles from Wissant on the coast road. The food was exceptional and especially the fruit de mer. Together with Robert, Gertie and Diana we went for lunch. Gertie and Robert indulged in two enormous bowls of moules, Diana in a very large plate of fruit de mer topped by a large lobster, and Nancy and I ate smoked salmon. The white wine was cool and smooth and the meal taken outside in the sunshine lasted some hours. This was living at its best.

Each night at the Normandy hotel we have our after dinner coffee outside. Robert and I have a cognac and as a ritual Robert gives a sugar lump dipped in cognac to the girls. This has been a repeated joke but Gertie rebelled and insists on her own cognac. It may sound silly but we do have fun.

Chapter 14

Visiting Professorships

My first visiting professorship was to the University of British Columbia in Vancouver in 1977. The invitation was initiated by Dr David Garrow who had trained in radiology at St Mary's Hospital, some years before me, David had been a Scottish junior golf champion, but sadly had contracted poliomyelitis affecting his legs and necessitating leg irons. He still played golf at a high level and flew his own aeroplane. His major contribution to medicine was his invention of the Garrow Box. This was a table on which the patient lay and beneath which was a box containing film cassettes, spring loaded. Following the injection of a radio-opaque dye into one of the major blood vessels, the box with its cassettes could be moved to predetermined positions and films taken in sequence following the flow of the dye in the blood vessels. Thus the vessel under investigation could be visualized. The main use was in the blood vessels of the abdomen and legs. Like many good inventions this was simple, cheap and durable. It was used world wide before more sophisticated equipment became available. These investigations demonstrated the exact diagnosis and extent of the damage to the blood vessels. So the operative treatment could be planned meticulously as never before. The techniques for introducing the dyes were devised and performed by radiologists and developed remarkably over the decades since the 1950s. These have led to many complex diagnostic and treatment procedures performed today.

I learnt some sharp lessons on this first professorship. I had agreed to see patients as well as lecture and give tutorials. I was unaware how difficult it is to use unfamiliar equipment for complex procedures in a strange environment, and for the operator, the assistant and the nurse to perform procedures when they haven't worked together before. I'd heard stories about mishaps concerning visiting consultants but hadn't learnt the lesson myself. I learnt it on this trip and my performance was less impressive than I wished. I learnt another lesson. I usually lighten my lectures with an occasional funny story. This works well at home in the United Kingdom, but in Canada was met with stony silence. This affected my confidence. The young doctors had a different sense of humour or perhaps didn't expect humour in a serious lecture. Perhaps I tried too hard. When the audience is unresponsive, I overplay my hand. It took three weeks before I got any response. In the meantime I suffered.

However my stay at Vancouver General Hospital was enjoyable. The medicine practised there was good, but each unit seemed to act in isolation. At the time this could have been the fault of the Department of Radiology, but the result was I didn't get to any combined meetings and made little or no contact with the other medical departments. The equipment in the department was basic in 1977 and this surprised me. The equipment for complex procedures was up to date as was the equipment in the private department. Patients were frequently subjected to a multiplicity of tests which often overlapped in their diagnostic value.

Some years later I saw this again when I lectured in the University of Southern California. One reason for this is the high incidence of claims for medical negligence. Under these threats of litigation such a multitude of tests is understandable. Less understandable is that with the system of payment in both Canada and the United States more tests generate more income to the department. There was and perhaps still is a strong emphasis on cost effectiveness across the Atlantic, which has come now to our shores. It distresses hospital administrators that in the United Kingdom the doctors are more interested in clinical effectiveness than cost effectiveness.

One of the last cases I saw during my time at Vancouver General was a surgical emergency. A young man, a professional football player, had an argument with his wife at breakfast. He drove to his training ground in a temper. He then had an argument with his football coach. He drove away in a temper and crossing a bridge at 100 mph hit the rigid spar at one end. Not wearing a seat belt he was severely injured. He had multiple fractures and was unconscious. He was in a state of shock with a low blood pressure and a weak pulse. There were signs of bruising over his chest. It was difficult to resuscitate him and his blood pressure continued to fall. The possibility that he had a tear in his aorta (the main large blood vessel coming out of the heart) seemed high. To confirm this it was necessary to place a tube in the aorta and inject a radio-opaque dye and get a radiograph of the artery. The tube was inserted and the dye injected. When the film was examined the dye was in the right position but a tear couldn't be seen. Part of the problem was that the bone of the spine was overlapping the artery and prevented adequate visualization. If there was a tear then a leakage of the dye should be seen. At the time, before more sophisticated equipment became available a photographic method of blocking out the bone was possible. This was done and the tear with the leakage was seen. At any time a catastrophic 'blow out' could occur with certain death. He was immediately brought to the theatre and an operation to close the tear was performed. He recovered and eventually left hospital. Today there is a technique called Digital Subtraction Angiography which can show blood vessels free from the overlying bone and this has been a major advance in diagnostic methods.

I brought copies of these films with me to London and used them in lectures for years They illustrated the value of radiological assessment leading to successful surgery.

In Vancouver Nancy and I had a suite in a hotel where we catered for ourselves. It was comfortable with a double bedroom, a sitting room and a kitchen. In the sitting room there was a large window looking out on Vancouver bay. We watched seaplanes land and take off; not something we could see in London. When I returned from the hospital in the evening we watched ice hockey on the television. I became addicted and looked forward to seeing favourite teams playing. Nancy loved her freedom in Vancouver and had no domestic responsibilities. She walked in the city, and in the park by the bay. She spent time in the library, reading the history of Canada and its people and visited the shops. She told friends then and subsequently that we had a working holiday. I worked while she had a holiday! She never told them however that I wouldn't or even couldn't go without her. Nancy calms my constant anxiety.

While we were away my eldest daughter, Siobhan, had a loan of Nancy's mini car. We had a letter from her:

> Dear Mother and Father,
>
> I've just been reading D.H. Lawrence and he makes the point that there are more important things in life than a passion for possessions. He says it is a small mind that holds material values in any importance. I certainly believe that and no doubt you do too.
>
> By the way, I've just crashed the car and it's a write off.
>
> Your loving daughter,
>
> Siobhan.

I saw very little of Canada while I was in Vancouver, as most of my time was spent in the hospital. Vancouver itself was beautiful, built around the bay with snow capped mountains as a backcloth. It was possible to swim or fish and then go up the mountains to ski on the same day. I knew I had a cousin living in Canada, but to my surprise she lived in Vancouver only a few hundred yards from our hotel. I hadn't known that before going . She and her husband entertained us and drove us into the mountains in their large convertible car.

We also got to Vancouver Island for a weekend. The scenery on the island is magnificent with woods and many beaches. The quality of life was very attractive and almost Victorian compared to the mainland. We stayed with a delightful couple, Monty Wright and his wife. Monty, a heavily built man with a neat Van Dyke beard, had been a fighter pilot in the Royal Air Force during World War Two. He was one of the first Canadian volunteers. He and I had mutual friends who had also been fighter pilots. Monty was the curator of the museum in Victoria, the capital of the island. We were entertained enthusiastically, including a visit to the museum.

There we saw reconstructions of Indian villages complete with wax figures of remarkable quality. There were also reproduced saloon bars and gold mines. Totem poles of varying tribes were displayed all beautifully carved. We had a delightful weekend only marred by my developing a rageing toothache which necessitated the removal of a tooth subsequently.

Nancy when walking around Vancouver felt she missed something and wasn't quite sure what it was. One night she said, 'I miss old stone walls which go back hundreds of years. I miss old European history. Every wall and every building is new'. I regret I hadn't noticed but when she said it – I did.

We returned to London refreshed in mind but a little tired in body.

My second Professorship was to the University of Queensland in Australia. I was given a first class ticket and told I could change it for two tourist class if I wished. I did. Nancy and I stayed in the Visiting Professor's Lodge in Brisbane. The invitation came from Professor Hiram Baddeley. Hiram had trained in radiology at St Mary's Hospital and I had taught him. He was an excellent radiologist who after his training took a registrar's post in Bristol where his chief was Professor Sir Howard Middlemiss. Howard was a legend in radiology and travelled throughout the underdeveloped countries bringing his skills to a multitude of hospitals. He taught and equipped departments of radiology world wide. He also arranged to send members of his own team on secondment to work and teach in these hospitals. Hiram, at Howard's request, worked in Africa before taking the chair in Brisbane.

While I was in Brisbane, Hiram's book on radiology was published. We had a champagne celebration. During this period Hiram travelled frequently to China to establish a hospital with Chinese doctors. This was a time when communication between China and the West was far from good, and his work was all the more remarkable for that.

I had decided before taking this professorship to confine myself to lecturing and giving tutorials. As a result it was more successful than my first. The young Australian medical students and post graduate doctors had a different culture to those in the United Kingdom. They were less reluctant to question and less intimidated by authority. You had to prove your worth and justify yourself daily. This was no bad thing. With more time available I was able to attend combined clinical meetings where I could make a modest contribution and indeed where I learnt much. This proved to be a most enjoyable trip.

Brisbane was an interesting town with a good climate. The shopping was good and they sold shirts for giants. With my increasing girth this was an advantage. The people were hospitable and we were invited to many homes. I was asked to give the speech at the Brisbane Annual Medical Dinner. I prepare after dinner speeches carefully and am aware that mostly people wish to be entertained. I invariably include some serious points in an effort not simply to be known as a comic.

However on that night I selected what I thought were my funniest Irish jokes. The dinner was excellent and the room packed. I only knew the few doctors from the hospital, the others were strangers. It's remarkable how quickly one knows when a speech isn't going well. That was such a night. To my horror, each Irish story was met with silence interrupted by an occasional laugh which only served to emphasize my failure and increase my embarrassment. After dinner I was introduced to many of the audience in the bar.

'Oscar, I'd like you to meet Dr O'Brien.'

'This is Dr Kelly.'

'Dr Sean Byrne is a local general practitioner. He always supports our annual dinner.'

The place was full of Irish doctors, descended from Irish immigrants. They thought I was 'taking the mickey' out of the Irish. What surprised me was they didn't recognize my Irish accent. With regard to after dinner speeches I protect my ego by thinking – you can't win 'em all.

There was a weekend free and we decided to see something of the Australian outback. A travel agent advised us to go to a nature camp in a rain forest called Binna Burra. We boarded the camp bus on a Friday evening, full of excitement, but not knowing what to expect. After some hours drive we arrived at the camp and signed in.

They weren't interested in our full names but merely wrote Nancy and Oscar, and as such were introduced to everyone. Nancy and I, old fashioned in these things, took some time to get used to the informality which has become so commonplace. We had a log cabin sitting on stilts high among the trees. It was beautiful and something entirely new to us. There was a sitting room with a large full length window looking into the forest and miles of trees, a double bedroom and a modern bathroom. The prize feature was a veranda which was virtually in the branches.

Birds were all around us, including colourful parakeets. On the open field of the camp we saw kangaroos hopping about.

Breakfast was in a large log cabin and was self service. We sat at any table of our choice and shared the room with about forty or fifty men, women and children. We didn't know what was to happen after breakfast but weren't left in doubt for long.

While we ate a member of the camp staff came to us.

'You can choose whatever activity you'd like today, but we've arranged a walk'.

'That's great. How far will you walk?'

'About twenty miles.'

'My God, we're over fifty and not used to walking such distances. We couldn't do it.'

'Well never mind. We have a party going abseiling. You can join them. The cliffs are quite small.'

'We've never abseiled and couldn't do that.'

'Oh dear, there is another party going horse riding.'

'I can do that but my wife doesn't ride.'

'This is difficult. Well you can go out on your own into the forest. We'll give you a map, a billy can with some tea leaves and sandwiches.

You can get water in the forest. Don't worry if you get lost, we'll send a search party for you if you're not back by dark. Stick to the route marked on the map.'

We got the map and haversacks and set off into the forest with some anxiety. The first thing we noticed was the strange noises. The one I'll never forget was the call of the whip birds. They are so well named and the shrill repeated call was hypnotic. I got the impression they were looking at us, calling us in and laughing at the same time.

The only water we found was a huge waterfall on the other side of a ravine impossible to get to without abseiling down the side of a cliff. This was impossible for us, so we ate dry sandwiches. I watched the route carefully. Although they told me if I followed the route marked on the map we would go in a circle and end up back at the camp, I wasn't too sure. So I made marks in the ground and on trees in case we had to go back the way we came. We seemed to walk forever. Ironically it could have been twenty miles; it certainly felt like twenty miles. We had started at 9.30 a.m. and arrived back at 4.30 p.m. I was wearing a pair of light brown city suede shoes totally unsuitable for walking in a rain forest. If only I'd known, I could have bought some walking boots. We arrived back bedraggled, starving, thirsty and exhausted. The campers smiled.

'Did you see any snakes?'

'Snakes! No, should we have?'

'Well, this is the waking season for snakes.'

I was glad I hadn't known that. Following the evening meal they held a barn dance. We saw them dancing, some with children on their shoulders. Unfit to go and still exhausted we crawled painfully to our cabin in the trees. We felt old, very very old. Like my shoes we were more suited to walking in Oxford Street.

On the Sunday we just lazed until lunch. At lunch we met a charming husband and wife, whose names I've forgotten. They could even have been Bruce and Sheila but I doubt that. They were about our age, and started the conversation.

'How are you getting back to Brisbane?'

'We're taking the camp bus.'

'You needn't do that. We're going to Brisbane and can give you a lift.'

'That would be lovely, thank you.'

'I've got an old Volvo which is the best car I've ever had. We've travelled all over Australia in it and it's never let me down. I'm so proud of it.'

After lunch we all climbed aboard the car and headed out into the deserted outback.

After an hour or so the Volvo came to a halt and couldn't be restarted. We were in the middle of nowhere. Our new friend was devastated. He lifted the bonnet and fiddled but with no success. I'm useless with engines and was no help to him. I wandered off the road into the bush for a few yards. He yelled, 'Come back. There may be snakes in there.'

I came back quickly but again thought of our walk through the rain forest the previous day.

After about half an hour a car came along the road and stopped. The occupant tried his skills at starting the car but also failed. Our friend said, 'Could you give me a lift to the nearest house and I'll phone for help?'

'Certainly I will, but I don't know where there is a house around here. We could drive for miles.'

They drove off and we remained by the car in some anxiety. After another half an hour a second car stopped and the driver asked if he could help. Told the story he offered to take us with him. It was tempting but we thought we'd better wait for our friend to return: his wife wouldn't think of any other possibility!

An hour later a large pick-up truck appeared with our friend and a mechanic. He couldn't fix the car, so it was towed for miles to the garage and we proceeded in the truck to Brisbane. All in all it was a weekend to remember.

I was invited to lecture in Perth on the other side of Australia before returning to London. The trip by plane took, as far as I remember, over four hours. Flying over the Great Victoria Desert, I was aware of the enormous size and sparseness of Australia.

Perth is a small town and at the time seemed like a frontier town. It was very beautiful sitting on the Black Swan River, close to the coast. The weather was idyllic and the vegetation tropical. We were met by an English radiologist who had resigned his consultant post in England to settle in Perth. He brought us to his house for tea after we'd settled into the hotel. He knew at the time I was on the Council of the Royal College of Radiologists in England and an examiner for the Fellowship of the College. He lost no time in telling me he thought the Royal College of Radiologists was a useless institution and that the Fellowship of the College was a valueless qualification. He then enlarged on his poor opinion of radiologists in the United Kingdom. To say the least I was astounded at his opinion and more so to give it to a Visiting Professor. It wasn't a great beginning to my visit to Perth.

I gave my lecture which the audience received well, and Nancy and I were invited to dinner at the prestigious Freemantle Yacht Club. Our teatime friend and his wife said, 'The dinner is informal, so don't dress up.'

To be informal I wore a blazer, flannels and my Garrick tie. When my friend and his wife picked us up wearing shorts and open necked shirts, she looked disparagingly at me and said, 'Oh, how pretty.'

If it was meant to make me feel uncomfortable, it failed. At dinner the guests were dressed as we were.

Nancy has a lovely memory of Perth, sitting under palm trees by the river watching the black swans glide past. You may appreciate my memories are different.

Chapter 15

Sydney

I was invited to Sydney, Australia, as Visiting Professor. It was our first trip to Sydney and our impression at the airport was disappointing. The flight had been long and we were tired. Perhaps it was just an off day. A large number of planes arrived within the one hour and renovations were being made at the airport. We had difficulty finding the luggage carousel as did a number of confused and irritated passengers who jostled and pushed amid an enormous din. We were unable to find a baggage trolley. By trial and error we found the carousel but had to wait a long time for the bags to appear. We then had a problem getting a taxi as the queue was enormous and the taxis appeared slowly. It was hot. At this low ebb I asked myself why I had agreed to make the trip at all. Nancy was silent and I knew she was exhausted. We felt better when we arrived at the flat in which we were to stay.

It was owned by Professor Janet McCredie and was in Darling Point overlooking Sydney Harbour. Janet was staying in a hotel in Sydney where she was organizing a radiological conference. The flat was lovely and the view wonderful. Each morning a helicopter took off from a house across the harbour. It returned each evening and the occupant to our amusement left the helicopter and immediately watered his flowers. Janet's flat opened onto a well kept lawn in which there was a swimming pool, beyond which the harbour sea lapped against the wall. What a dream place in which to live.

I settled into lecturing and attending clinical meetings. One of my colleagues said as this was our first visit to Sydney his wife Jackie would show us some of the sights.

Jackie arrived in a large Australian car. She was dressed in white slacks, white blouse and a pink cardigan. Hanging from her neck were large brown beads. She was slim, average in height and had auburn hair. As we introduced ourselves I was drawn to her dark, deepset brown eyes, which shimmered and glowed, seducing me totally. Her charm was captivating and difficult to resist. I thought she was either saint or devil but it didn't seem to matter which. Smiling at us she said, 'Now let me show you Sydney and I can play both tourist and guide.'

We set off on a wonderful day of sightseeing and fun. We began at a fish market where Jackie bantered and bartered with the fishmongers amid much laughter and got the fish for her evening meal. We drove around the harbour area dominated by the heavily arched Sydney bridge, close to the Royal Australasian College of Radiologists. The magnificent opera house was even more impressive than in the photographs I'd seen. The impression of billowing sails was strong and beautiful. I was surprised that the roof consisted of individual self-cleaning tiles, not obvious on the usual photographs in brochures.

The harbour was busy with boats passing to and fro, including brightly coloured sailing boats. The sea was a moving platform of colour, full of mirrors of reflecting sun, jumping and dancing to greet our excited eyes. We didn't linger long in one spot, but drove on in constant expectation of a new delight around the corner. We saw Rock Island and suffered awhile with the convicts isolated on it in bygone days for further punishment. Sharks prevented any escape. In contrast we saw Point Piper, one of Sydney's most fashionable suburbs, with exotic houses reaching to the sea. Nelson Rock and its Surf Club, where the waves are said to be dangerous, was impressive, but frightened me by the need to have a shark-proof net. It is referred to as Shark Bay. We had lunch in the Benelong Restaurant in the Opera house. The sights were wonderful but came alive through the passion of Jackie in showing them and in a strange way she became part of every building, every bridge, every bay and every man and woman we met.

She was tireless and her vivacity and excitement set Nancy and me alight. I thought there never was such radiance in one woman and years later as I write these words, I can still feel her vigour and bewitchment.

As we left her that evening I had to know what gave her that quality, that spirit, that fire.

'Why are you so much fun to be with and what gave you this zest for life?'

'I've been born again.'

I prepared myself for an evangelical eulogy but she had a mischievous smile which made me suspect another answer.

'I was dying with kidney failure but I've had a kidney transplant and I'm alive and life is wonderful.'

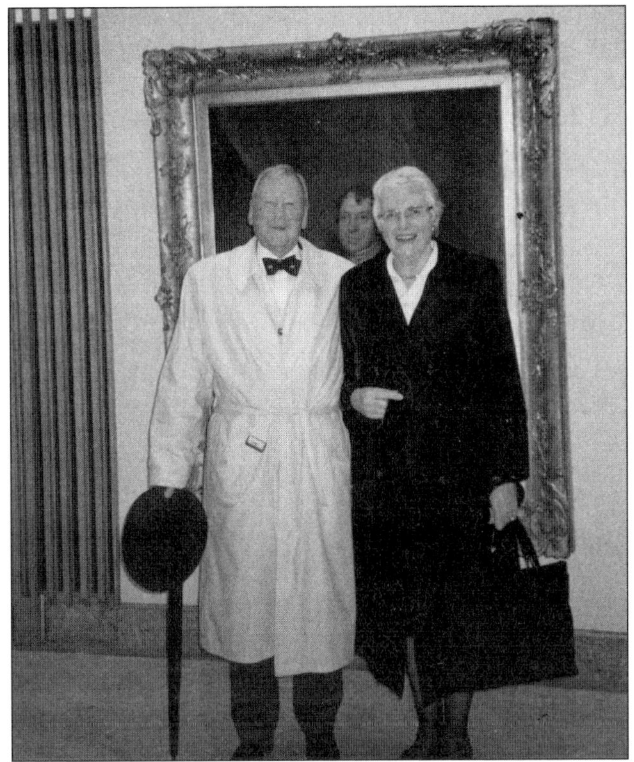

The author with Professor Janet McCredie

She made me think again of the value of medicine, the value of research and the many disappointments as the profession struggled to perfect transplantations. I had witnessed these efforts and had also been disheartened in their early days.

Jackie found while in hospital she could paint. She had talent and held an exhibition in Paris shortly after I returned home. I always regret I didn't see it.

Three Australian Professors of Radiology trained in the Department of Radiology at St Mary's Hospital in Paddington, Professors Hiram Baddeley, John Palmer and Janet McCredie.

Janet McCredie studied medicine in Sydney but came to London to do her post graduate training in radiology in 1960. She was the first female trainee in the Department of Radiology in St Mary's Hospital. She had an enquiring mind and a direct and confident manner. When I taught her she repeatedly asked, 'Why do you say that, Dr Craig? Have you proof for your statement?' Until then, in the early 1960s, no trainee had questioned my teaching. I was now having to prove facts I'd been taught and had been teaching for years. Janet made me aware I hadn't scientific proof for many of the accepted theories in medicine. She certainly kept me on my toes. The calibre of Janet can be illustrated by the story of her visit to Russia at the height of the cold war. When leaving Moscow at the airport she had to sign a document concerning currency. The Russian official also had to sign it and borrowed her pen. After signing he put her pen in his pocket and walked away. Janet said, 'You've got my pen. Can I have it back, please?'

He walked on behind the counter to another room. Janet turned to another official standing nearby, 'That man has taken my pen and I want it back.' The other passengers watching the events said,

'Janet, the plane is leaving. Don't make a fuss. Leave the pen. Just come on.'

'No, I won't move until I get my pen back.'

She stood firm and refused to move. Some minutes passed. The atmosphere was tense. The man was sent for and returned the pen.

At the time the relationship between Russia and the West was touchy. I'm a coward – I would have left the pen.

I reminded Janet of this incident quite recently and she said, 'I've always regretted that I missed an opportunity. When he returned the pen, I should have given it to him.'

I see her point and what a triumph it would have been.

Toward the end of 1971 Janet was asked by an obstetric colleague to look at twelve malformed babies. Five of them were thalidomide victims. She was asked to say from the deformities of the bones seen on radiographs which cases were due to thalidomide. She decided to study the thalidomide cases and started by getting the particular radiographic examinations she wanted. Although the bones were short and deformed with joint deformities as well, she concluded early on that the X-ray features were not consistent with a disease affecting bones and joints directly. There had to be some other explanation. She referred to the text books and looked at diseases that might cause similar joint deformities. She found a set of diseases which affected the sensory nerves with joint deformities similar to those in the thalidomide cases. These diseases were leprosy, diabetes, syphilis and a disease of the spinal cord called syringomyelia. The disorders were due to nerve damage, i.e. neurotrophic. Janet came to the conclusion that the sensory nerves of the developing child, the embryo, were damaged by thalidomide leading to the deformity of the limbs. The damage to the nerves happened as early as the first few weeks and the site of the damage was the neural crest. It was this nerve damage that led to the failure of the bones to grow and led to the joint deformities in addition. This was a theory new to medicine.

Professor McCredie flew to England to see Professor Howard Middlemiss in Bristol. He had seen many cases of neurotrophic disease in adults who had bone and joint deformities but in fully developed limbs. Howard was impressed by Janet's theory and encouraged her to do further research. She visited Queen Mary's Hospital Roehampton where she had access to one hundred cases.

She said, 'the same answers kept emerging.' She wrote a paper on her theory for publication in *Clinical Radiology*, the Journal of the Royal College of Radiologists. The paper included the five cases from her obstetric colleague. The paper firmly fixed the site of damage from thalidomide at the neural crest.

In 1977 Professor McCredie was awarded the Twining Medal of the Royal College of Radiologists of the United Kingdom for her research. In 1979, acknowledging her authorship she was awarded the Peter Bancroft Prize for Post Graduate Research by the University of Sydney. She was described as being well known for her development of the neural crest theory to explain the origin of many types of congenital abnormality. Also in 1979 she was awarded a Doctorate by the University of Sydney for her thesis on 'Neural Crest Defects'. In 1983 she was awarded the Singer Medal for Research by the United States of America. In 1991 the University of Sydney awarded her the Lowenthal Medal for her scientific contribution to medicine. In 1994 Professor McCredie was awarded the AM, i.e. Member of the Order of Australia for services to Diagnostic Radiology and Medical Research.

Janet has reported on five hundred British infants born deformed due to thalidomide and four thousand in West Germany where she has worked with Professor Hans Willert.

I was elected President of the Harveian Society of London in January 2002. As President I had to choose the Harveian Lecturer for 2002. I wished to choose someone worldwide who had contributed original work to medicine, in the tradition of Harvey. It isn't surprising that I choose Professor Janet McCredie. No fee is attached to this lecture and no expenses are paid, it is considered purely an honour to be asked. Janet with great enthusiasm accepted the invitation and flew to London.

She gave the lecture 'Ariadne's Thread and the Labyrinth of Congenital Abnormalities', on Wednesday 9th January 2002. Professor Hans Willert flew from Germany to be present. Many distinguished radiologists and neurologists attended and the lecture was a great success.

I was proud I had taught her the early steps in her career in Clinical Radiology.

Professor John Palmer, an Englishman, also trained in the Department of Radiology at St Mary's Hospital and then emigrated to Australia. He was responsible along with Dr John Cashman, an Australian radiologist, for assessing the use of dyes (contrast media), used for injections into the blood stream for radiological investigations. The assessment was indicated because these media have side effects which are often serious, and newer safer contrast media had been developed. However these new media, known as low osmolar media, were substantially more expensive. They would put a financial strain on Health Authorities and especially in Great Britain would have serious consequences for the funding of the Health Service. However the problem was world wide. John Palmer and John Cashman investigated these chemicals and their effect on patients undergoing a variety of radiological investigations with one or the other. They produced a paper of sound scientific and clinical value. As a result of their findings it became policy in Australia only to use the more expensive low osmolar contrast media. I agree with this decision. Such a policy was not adopted in the United Kingdom at the time. Advice was sought by the Royal College of Radiologists from two radiologists expert in the field of contrast media, Professor Ronald Grainger and Professor Peter Dawson. Criteria were published indicating in which cases low osmolar contrast should be used. I feel however we have merely postponed adopting the policy indicated by the Australian investigation.

John Palmer and Janet McCredie continue to practise in Australia. Hiram Baddeley returned to London where he holds a consultant post.

Two further professors trained in the department at St Mary's, Aghiad Al Kutoubi who holds a chair in Beirut and Graham Cherryman who has the chair of radiology in Leicester.

Chapter 16

The National Health Service

I believe the United Kingdom in establishing a National Health Service in 1948 gave the world an example of how the health of any nation should be cared for. In no country should any individual be denied adequate medical treatment for lack of money. I've always been grateful that my major practice was in the Health Service. I had private patients in the Lindo Wing of St Mary's Hospital and am not opposed to private practice, but regret it is necessary under any circumstances. I believe the remuneration in medical practice should be sufficiently good within the NHS to offset any desire to practise privately. This is an Utopian ideal and I'll never see it. During my long service in the NHS I've seen how it works, in general practice, as a surgeon in my junior hospital days and as a consultant in clinical radiology and Director of the Department of Radiology. My active years spanned from 1950 to 1992 and even in retirement I've been close to my colleagues in hospital practice. I feel entitled to question why in these days the ideals of the NHS are not being realized, and why the morale of the profession is so low. It's not possible to lay the blame at a single door. The responsibility must be shared between successive governments, the medical fraternity, lay management and apathy on the part of medical bodies such as the British Medical Association, the Medical Royal Colleges and even the General Medical Council. I'm aware the NHS is a bottomless pit financially and also that throwing money into it will not solve the problems, helpful though it may be. I also fear that as we cannot meet the demands on the NHS, government measures move us closer to a two-tiered health service. When I began in general practice the National Health Service had only been in operation for two years. It was fifty three years ago and consequently I've seen enormous changes. Some of these changes have been beneficial but many detrimental to both patients and doctors.

In general practice in 1950 surgeries were packed and it was not unusual to have as many as forty patients to see at both a morning and evening surgery. Many just needed repeat prescriptions which took little time but they were seen and this served as a follow up. There can be a danger in repeating prescriptions without seeing the patient. There was no appointment system and patients often waited for two hours. No specific length of time was allotted to each patient with the doctor, but each was given the time necessary to meet the presenting problem. It was important that the patient didn't feel rushed and the benefit was a relaxed atmosphere allowing the patient to communicate better with the doctor and vice versa. Frequently the patient needed time to reveal a hidden fear. There was time to enquire about the patient's family. This was part of one's duty as a family doctor. Understanding the circumstances in which patients lived helped when problems arose that affected the whole family. Surgeries were long and evening surgeries seldom finished before 8 p.m.. Home visits were common and I remember days, in the winter especially, when I did twenty home visits. Night calls were not unusual and there was no deputizing service. Life was full and interesting. There was little abuse of the doctor's time. In the 1950s the relationship between the doctor and his patient was excellent.

Much has changed since then. General practitioners are better informed and attend more clinical meetings to keep up to date with medical developments. Appointment systems have been introduced and computerized records add to the overall efficiency.

It is no longer necessary to wait two hours to get a repeat prescription. Some changes are less satisfactory. Although there is less waiting, many appointments are scheduled for ten minutes. I have heard often, 'the doctor was very busy and in a rush'. There is less time to really communicate. Doctors make fewer home visits and often night calls are done by a deputizing service. Patients dislike being seen by a deputizing doctor, who knows little about them or their circumstances. Communication between the deputizing doctor and the practice isn't always satisfactory. It can be difficult to monitor subtle changes in the patient's condition when seen by different doctors.

As doctors become more technical the ability to hold hands seems to be fading. There are times when all the doctor can do is to hold a patient's hand.

Compassionate hand holding is an essential part of good doctoring. This trend is not confined to general practice. In hospital practice technological advances in diagnosis and treatment have been remarkable. Patients are living longer and the quality of life has been improved. I am anxious however that the machine may become the physician. Communication skills and empathy with the patient have not kept pace with the advance in technology. I have heard the following conversation, 'How am I doing doctor?'

'Don't ask me until the reports of the tests are back.'

There is an emphasis today on informed consent to investigations and treatments.

This is an advance and every patient should indeed know why particular procedures are being recommended. It is sad that even with this emphasis informed consent is not always obtained. This can often be due to the patient's confusion or inability to understand, but it is the doctor's duty to appreciate this and deal with it. It is a problem today that patients' expectations regarding treatments are often too high and if disappointed they suspect someone has erred. This can lead to litigation and the possibility of litigation is now a fact of medical practice as never before. In turn this leads to the practice of defensive medicine where more tests are performed than are necessary. To omit a possible test makes the physician more vulnerable even though he or she may think it unnecessary. In some ways progress is threatened as fewer doctors are willing to undertake innovative procedures.

Since I entered the NHS fifty three years ago the mutual trust between the doctor and the patient has declined significantly. Mutual respect has also suffered. Is it not disgraceful that the staff of accident and emergency departments need police protection.

I have heard complaints about paternalism on the part of doctors, surprisingly not from patients, but from health service committees of varying kinds, and I have read of it in various medical publications. However I believe that the public and the medical profession don't suffer from too much medical paternalism but too often from a lack of it. It is a doctor's duty to act at all times in the best interests of his patient, and this may sometimes necessitate paternalism. I appreciate that this must be accompanied by the doctor's awareness of his accountability.

The General Medical Council issued a publication in 1999, 'Seeking patient's consent: the ethical considerations'. In it the GMC stated, 'It is for the patient not the doctor to determine what is in the patient's own interests.' I appreciate that it is the patient who in the long run must decide to accept or reject the advice given, but it is my experience that few patients are gifted in knowing which of many alternative investigations and treatments are in his or her best interests. Neville Goodman writing in the *Journal of the Royal Society of Medicine*, February 2000, wrote 'what is the point of five years of medical school, a more intense than ever postgraduate medical education and all the rest, if the presumption at the end is that the doctor knows no more or no better than the patient.' I believe it is the moral duty of the doctor to advise the patient what is in his or her best interests. To put this burden on the patient is wrong and merely 'passes the buck'. At best it is a shared decision, but the doctor must take the lead and the responsibility.

As things are in the NHS today it doesn't support the patient's confidence if the doctor has to delay treatment or investigations because of the deficiency in technological aids such as CT scanners or Magnetic Resonance imagers. There is insufficient staff and the waiting lists are too long. It is devastating to the patient to have an operation cancelled because the wards or the operating theatres are closed. It also does little for the morale of the medical profession who in the long run have to cope with the disappointed and frustrated patient. Added to this the doctor has to deal with too much lay management, too many committees and too much paper work, all of which take the doctor away from clinical work. The result is that the compassionate role of the doctor may be lost.

These thoughts may be a generalization and thankfully the majority of doctors are compassionate and conscientious and there is much good in the working of the NHS. However I feel that in the present climate doctors will have to work hard to regain the mutual confidence that existed between them and their patients in the past. Mutual confidence is an essential to practise good medicine. I'm an optimist that it will return in due time.

I have mentioned that doctors do not take easily or kindly to management. The management of the National Health Service has changed enormously since I qualified. In an article published in the *Sunday Times* of 1st June 2003 it stated the number of managers and support staff in the NHS was 269,080 while there are 266,170 qualified nurses and 100,319 doctors of which only 62,476 are employed in hospitals. Since 1995 the number of senior managers has increased by 48% and the number of managers by 24%. But the number of qualified nurses has increased by only 7.8%. The figures speak for themselves and surely to any reasonable mind this is a ridiculous state of affairs. As the government produces targets to achieve it produces more managers when what is needed is more doctors and nurses.

When I was appointed a hospital consultant in 1963 the hospital was led by a strong medical committee which had an elected medical chairman. The hospital administration was in the hands of a House Governor and to help him he had a small team. The matron also had a significant administrative role. The House Governor attended the medical committee meetings and carried out the wishes of the medical committee, but also advised the committee when he thought the wishes needed modification. It was a very healthy relationship which worked well. We now have career health service managers with enormous staffs, and they don't have the same relationship with the medical committee as previously. Some editorials appeared in the *British Medical Journal* of 22nd March 2003, which addressed the problem between doctors and managers. They referred to the tension that existed between them. It was even suggested that patients are best served by a tension between the two. I doubt that. It must be recognized however that doctors are not good managers, but know what is best for their patients. The editorial stated, 'if managers suddenly became preoccupied with the needs of an individual patient, irrespective of the consequences for others or for their budget, then the health system would collapse.' I'm not sure I totally agree with this. Various points are made, 'Doctors think first about their individual patients, managers think first about organizations. For any hospital or primary care trust to succeed, it will need both kinds of thinking.' Some truths are stated, 'Doctors are also uneasy with being led: they are too individualistic; managers also tend to be more comfortable with working in teams; many doctors are too inclined to dominate teams.'

It is suggested that a solution might be to improve the quality of health service managers or possibly make managers think and behave like doctors or vice versa.

The overall message was that managers and doctors could learn much from each other and must work more in harmony. Managers could benefit from being closer to patients and doctors need to think strategically.

It has been suggested that doctors could take a degree in management. I would be in favour of this. Many doctors might be happy to make a career in hospital administration and could take an MBA in the same way as a surgeon takes an FRCS or a physician an FRCP.

Perhaps well qualified medical managers might be successful in administration and whatever tensions exist might be less.

A further more far reaching article appeared in the same issue entitled, 'Doctors in chambers'. It suggested a possibility in the future is for doctors to operate independently from chambers, in the same fashion as barristers, and they would sell their services to hospitals.

This would indeed be a cataclysmic change.

Chapter 17

American Visitors

I'VE HAD MANY CARS in my lifetime and regret I've wasted too much money on them even though they have given me pleasure. In my young days they had to be second hand but eventually I graduated to new cars. When my four daughters were young Nancy persuaded me to buy a new blue Austin Cambridge Estate. I kept this car longer than most. My third daughter Finella, very young at the time, took a large bite out of the black plastic dashboard. This distressed me but I learnt to live with it. The car was heavy, slow but reliable and served us very well for all our needs. It had enormous chrome bumpers, and the tail gate opened down to provide a platform, excellent for picnics. It was a family friendly car and I think it was the last of the good Austins. A remarkable incident happened when we took this car to Ireland for a holiday. We drove to Glendalough, a tourist arca deep in the Wicklow mountains outside Dublin with a large lake surrounded by breathtaking undulating beauty. I drove the car into the car park where large boulders were used to mark off the spaces. We walked by the lake, had a picnic, visited the tourist shop and as was our custom, bought nothing. We were as relaxed as the Irish countryside and its inhabitants. We sauntered back to the car. I started the engine and put the car in gear and drove forward. I should have backed out, as the boulders were in front, and the car mounted them beautifully. It would go no further either forwards or back. It was stuck and the front was high in the air firmly fixed, with the back wheels on the ground. The car was now at an angle of some twenty or so degrees to the ground. Soon a crowd gathered and in their Irish fashion determined to be of help.

'Ah sure, you've got yourself into a bit of trouble there.'

'Yes, I think I have.'

'Now I don't think you could drive over those boulders.'

'No, I don't think I could.'

Another male voice came from the crowd.

'Might you try to go back the way.'

'I've tried that.'

'Might you be tryin' that again now?'

'I will.'

I tried and nothing happened. Another voice sounded.

'Are you sure you've it in reverse?'

'Yes I am.'

Another voice, 'It's not workin'.'

I heard them talking to each other.

'He's got a bit of trouble here. It's an English car.'

Another voice, 'What the hell difference does that make?'

'Sure I don't know, but it could.'

Still talking to each other, 'Sure they'll be here all night. Would they like some tea?'

I decided to try and get out and phone for help but at that moment a giant of a man who was standing at the back of the crowd silently watching walked forward, and mounted the boulders. He turned his back to the front of the car, steadied his feet, bent down and grasped the bumpers in his hands and lifted. The front of the car rose. The children in the back screamed and jumped out. The man moved back still holding the bumpers and deposited the car on the ground. The giant never spoke, never smiled but just turned and walked away. At first there was silence but then spontaneous applause broke out from the crowd followed by a cheer. The giant walked on and never looked back.

In the 1960s I went through a bad patch and needed to boost my ego. I saw a lovely Lancia Zagato sports car at the Motor Show. Shortly after that Nancy said, 'Your birthday is coming soon and although you are going to pay for it I've ordered that Lancia for you. I knew you wouldn't. Get it for your birthday.'

That car was the envy of the medical students. It was white, low slung and sexy. It was beautiful and eyecatching. One day, George Bonney, the orthopaedic surgeon was asked,

'Whose car is that?'

'Oh, that's Oscar Craig's image intensifier.'

It should not be so but that car made me feel better.

In the late 1970s in a moment of insanity I bought a second hand Bentley. It arrived at my home with a very large bouquet of flowers for Nancy. The salesman, smooth as smooth, delivered both personally with more flourish and élan than ever came with my other cars. We were suitably impressed and felt we had moved into another gear in our lifestyle. The car had a lovely elegant physiognomy; it was comfortable and impressive. Surprise, surprise – I was never happy with it. My decision hadn't considered the difficulty of parking and the problems of driving this enormous vehicle in London traffic. A dent or scratch would cost me thousands. Twelve miles to a gallon! The brakes were too soft and the tracking was never right.

One night as I approached it parked outside the hospital I saw it had a flat tyre. I was already fed up with the car. Any desire to have such a vehicle had gone forever.

I called the local garage. When the mechanic came I said, 'I'm quite unlucky with this car. I could do without it.'

He gave me a strange look and after a pause said quite sharply, 'I'd like to have some of your luck.'

His remark got to me. How right he was. I was chastened and thought what a prig I was. I've never forgotten him or the value of what he said.

However I couldn't go on driving it so I said to Nancy who at the time was driving a smart red Mini,

'Do you like the Bentley?'

'I love it.'

'OK. You can have it and I'll drive the Mini.'

Nancy did love driving that car. It was a joy to her to pick up the children from Wimbledon High School and a joy to go shopping in Cheam. The shopkeepers would carry her purchases to the car with some reflected pride and laugh and joke with her. They were disappointed when she walked and coming out of the shop had to put the purchases in the pram she was pushing.

I enjoyed the Mini and still think it a sensible car for town driving. However it has problems and it proved inadequate when I brought a visiting American VIP doctor home for tea to Cheam in it. He was from Texas and was over six foot tall and almost as broad. He had to roll down the window and lean his arm and shoulder out of the car to be able to sit in the seat. He looked at me rather strangely when he asked, 'Can we call for my wife.'

Not fully appreciating his strange look I replied, 'Of course, that will be delightful.'

We called for his wife at the Grosvenor House Hotel in Park Lane. I sat in the car while he went in to pick her up. When I saw them coming it was my turn to worry and look concerned. My heart missed several beats, for horror of horrors, she was bigger. We stood on the pavement and moved the front seats as for forward as possible and kept their backs folded down. She tried to get into the back seat head first. It was impossible. I advised her not to go head first but to back in with her enormous bottom going in first. We held both her hands as she slowly squeezed part of her bottom on to the seat and edged to the right. We still had her legs outside, so we lifted them up and pushed them in diagonally across the back. It was now difficult to get the backs of the front seats into position but we pushed them against her legs and feet. I thought it wise to get into the driving seat before her husband got in, as I expected some difficulty. The front seats were now too close to the dash board but we had to put up with that. Her husband, now slightly wiser, slid into his seat backside first with the door fully open. The car was listing to the right at this stage.

His enormous knees were just under his chin. Unfortunately, I had to get out again as he couldn't close the door. We left the window open again and I first gently but then firmly pushed the door. Eventually with his arm and shoulder out the window again I managed to close it. We started on the long drive to Cheam. There was little conversation on the way but I could hear them both breathing heavily. The car was not happy with this load and its listing significantly to the right made steering very difficult and with my arms forcibly pushed to my sides I couldn't manoeuvre freely. With this weight, when we stopped at traffic lights or queues the car couldn't pick up speed again. The journey accordingly was longer than usual and what took one and a half hours lengthened to two hours. When we arrived I thought they would fall out of the car, but when I opened the doors they didn't. I realized they were wedged in and couldn't move. I had to pull quite hard to get him out first and then we were joined by Nancy and the three of us managed with great difficulty to get his wife out, feet and legs first and then sliding her onto the drive. They were so red in the face and puffing you'd have thought they had walked the whole way. Later I thought that might have been easier.

When they were due to go back to town I told them I had a bigger car in the garage, but he said, 'If you have a phone we'll call for a cab.'

'I can show you the bigger car.'

'Doctor Craig, please don't do that. We'll call for a cab. It'll be easier.'

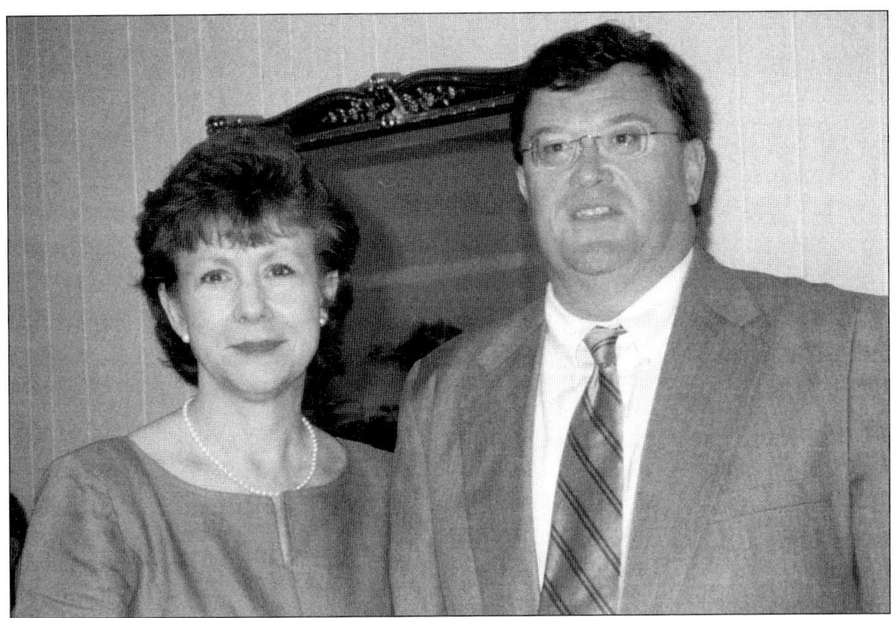

Dr and Mrs Frank Graybeal

They ordered a limousine. When this enormous car arrived they moved off waving enthusiastically. I've never seen or heard from them again.

We met two delightful Americans some years ago at a meeting of the Shadows, Frank and Nancy Graybeal. Ian Kerr had invited them as his guests to the Sunday lunch at his home in Haywards Heath. We were introduced to them just before we left for home and I was fascinated by their soft American drawl and wanted to find out more about them.

'Where are you from in America?'

'We live in North Carolina but come from South Carolina.' With a laugh he said, 'We sure is southern folk.'

'What are you doing in London?'

'Ah'm doin' a medical locum in the Brompton Hospital in Dr Kerr's department, and Nancy is just havin' a good time.'

'Where are you staying?'

'We've rented an apartment in Kensington.'

'Is this your first visit?'

'It sure is.'

I was attracted to both of them. Frank was medium in height but rotund and heavy. He had short black hair, wore spectacles and had a charming manner with a twinkle of devilment in his smile . When he spoke to you he gave you all his attention and looked directly into your eyes. I thought here is a man who is direct and honest. There is no pretence here. What you see is what you get! Nancy was pretty and slim. She had a laugh in her voice as she spoke and had lovely eyes which were also honest and direct. Her femininity was attractive and her gentle caring manner made you feel comfortable with her.

I wanted to see more of them and conscious of the impersonal nature of cities abroad wished to invite them home.

'Can you and Nancy come to dinner at our home next Thursday evening? By the way as there are two Nancys, we'll call my Nancy, Nancy B for Britain and your's Nancy A for America.'

'That sounds swell. Nancy A and ah would sure like to come to your home'.

'Great, come about 7.30. Take a train from Victoria station to Cheam and preferably one going through Hackbridge. That takes about half an hour. The train going through Norbury stops at so many stations in the south suburbs it's tedious and takes at least forty five minutes. We're about three minutes walk from Cheam village station.'

I drew for them a primitive map of the walk from the station.

We invited some local friends to join us for dinner. The dinner was hilarious. Frank turned out to be almost a caricature of an American Southerner. He was proud of his southern origins and made it clear he was not a Yankee. He believed in the heritage of southern gentlemen both in manners and attitudes. He and Nancy A captivated my guests from the moment of introduction.

'It's real good to meet you, Sir.' That was a winner.

'It sure is good to meet you Ma'am.' The ladies warmed to that.

During the dinner the talk came round to European wars and Frank looked at us and said in an earnest voice, 'Ah tell you de wah is not ova.'

The room fell silent at this and we all stared at Frank, not sure what war he was talking about, and had we heard him right. He repeated it in the silence, 'De wah is not ova. Those Yankees think it is, but I tell you de wah is not ova.' Seconds seemed like minutes as we sat thinking and then smiles broke out all around the table. Yes, we had heard right and Frank was talking about the American Civil War. This sentence has never died in our memories and when we think of Frank in Cheam we say, 'De wah is not ova.'

This may be said in jest, but there is a wealth of feeling behind the remark which speaks of a deep rooted emotion felt by Frank for the values of the southern states of America, southern people and their manners. He is aware of respect for family values and honesty in everything. He is proud of southern hospitality and critical of Yankee brashness, self interest and coarse behaviour. If there are good and admirable Northerners, Frank hates to admit it. I believe Frank would like to see the Civil War fought again, but would strive to see it had a different outcome!

Frank and Nancy A are anglophiles. This surprised us as we think standards in the British Isles are declining. Not so to them. They love London. They love the English countryside and especially Yorkshire. They have read all the James Herriot books and have seen all the television episodes. They buy the videos. On this first trip they visited Yorkshire and managed to see the filming of one of the episodes of the series. An added bonus was that James Herriot was there and they got him to autograph one of his books.

We took them to the Surrey County Show in Guildford. They came to Cheam and we piled into my car with all the necessary food, wine, walking sticks, raincoats and cloth caps. I made sure to pack the green wellington boots. We drove to Guildford, parked the car in the middle of a field with hundreds of others and made sure to mark in our minds where it was.

'The first thing to do is see the animals.'

'Great, we'll do that.'

We saw the cattle and marvelled at the variety of breeds. We smiled at the enormous size of the Charolais and the comparison with the tiny Dexters. We saw majestic thick necked large headed bulls whose androgenic features captivate Nancy B. We admired the Jacob sheep with their multiple horns and the long haired Angora breed.

The goats that took our fancy were the arrogant aristocratic Nubians. Next we toured the stalls and tents selling country crafts of every description. We saw walking sticks, knitwear, crockery, leather goods, wood carvings, silver, hats, coats, Barbours and imitation Barbours, good and at half the price. We paused to see pastries, jams, honey, farm wines, sausages and cheese, pickles and onions. We sampled some of the wines and cheese. We went into the flower tent where the two Nancys chatted over the exhibits and admired the prize winners' exhibitions.

Outside again we watched craftsmen making fences with intertwining ash branches and blacksmiths shoeing horses. It was lunch time. We walked back to the car having had the back of our hands stamped for re-entry.

Up went the folding table, on went the tablecloth, up went the folding chairs and on went the cutlery. Glasses were next and then filled with wine. The plates followed and soon were filled with a choice of ham, tomatoes, onions, coleslaw, cold fat sausages, small pork pies and chutney. This course was followed by cheese and a third glass of wine! It would be some time before driving home and if there was any doubt about my alcohol state, Nancy B would oblige.

On the way to the jumping enclosure after lunch we stopped to see the vintage cars. Frank and I love the nostalgic beauty of these vehicles for which there is no match on the roads today. We saw old Bentleys and Aston Martins but also beautiful production models, Sunbeam Talbots, Fords, Austins, Jaguars, Alfas and Citroens. There was one Bugatti and a very old Armstrong Siddeley.

On to the jumping enclosure with its special allure. Groomed and gallant the riders competed with grace, unmindful of the dangers of a fall, on horses prancing in anticipation, with flared nostrils and eager eyes. The pleasure of a clear round was greeted with applause and the disappointment of a fallen fence with groans. The spectators entered into the spirit of the competition as if it really mattered, as though they owned the horse, ridden by a relative. It was a compelling atmosphere.

Frank and Nancy A wallowed in the county scene.

It began to rain but the day was almost over. However Nancy A and Frank bought wellington boots which they still have so many years later. We drove home tired but well pleased. It had been a good day and our pleasure in the fair was enhanced by experiencing a familiar scene through the eyes of American visitors to whom this English country pursuit was new.

Some weeks later I phoned Frank, 'Nancy and I are going to Paris for the weekend.'

Frank didn't say anything for some seconds.

'Are you there, Frank?'

'Yes, Oscar, ah's thinkin'. Nancy A and ah would sure love to go to Paris.'

'Great, come with us. I'll book the flight and the hotel. Meet us at Terminal 2 in Heathrow on Friday night at the Air France counter. In case of problems I'll let you know the time and flight number.'

We left early on Friday evening and landed one hour later. As luck would have it Paris was having a heat wave. At first this pleased us. On the Saturday morning I decided Frank and Nancy A should see all the usual tourist attractions. This would take the whole day and part of Sunday. We were coming back late on Sunday night. So we set off to visit the Eiffel Tower, Notre Dame, the Left Bank for lunch. Musée D'Orsay, Sacre Coeur, major shops, Arc de Triomphe and the Champs Elysées. We took the Metro to the centre of Paris. At this stage Frank was already overhot and his heavy build added to the problem. He also had an assortment of cameras around his neck. Coming out of the train he said, 'Ah's used to heat but my Gad, this is somethin' else.'

We had to climb stairs coming out of the Metro and there were many. Frank was perspiring like I've never seen. His breathing became laboured as he dragged each foot up the stairway. He fell behind us but we waited at the top. When he appeared he was bent, both his back and his legs and the cameras were hitting his knees. There was pain all over his soaking face. He stood still for what seemed and age and then spoke, 'As ah came up, ah felt somethin' bangin' on my heels and it was my ass.'

Nancy A said, 'Frank, don't say such things.'

Nancy A is as delicate in temperament and speech as Frank is direct and blunt. Needless to say we all laughed and another choice saying entered our lives. Frank is indeed a colourful character.

The weekend was wonderful, the food and wine were good and both Frank and Nancy A loved Paris. However Frank said he felt more at home in London.

Chapter 18

North Carolina

When Frank and Nancy returned to America, the friendship continued by letter.

Soon we were getting invitations to holiday with them at their home in Fuquay-Varina in North Carolina. Fuquay-Varina is a small town close to Raleigh and by good fortune there is a direct flight from Gatwick. It couldn't be easier. The date was fixed and Frank met us at the airport in Raleigh, with his two children Meg and Russ.

My impression of America came from my visits to San Francisco, Chicago, New York, Los Angeles and Boston. It is a large country and Fuquay-Varina is a different America. It is however an America I've seen in the films. My first sensation on this trip was space, policemen with guns, large cars, enormous car parks and shopping centres, wide streets, baseball hats and jeans, trainer shoes and 'have a nice day'.

We drove a few miles to their colonial style house set in a pine forest. In the driveway sat three cars and two motor boats. There is a Jaguar, a sign of Frank's anglophile leanings, a multiple people vehicle in which we arrived, and which has a television set in the back, and a pick-up truck, an expression of the American male macho image.

'Why have you got a pick-up truck?'

'Every man sure needs a pick-up truck for huntin'.'

I thought I didn't need one in Cheam. Since that first visit Frank has added a convertible sports car and a Harley Davidson motor cycle.

The house sits in large grounds where there is also a swimming pool. The limits of the land are marked by pine trees and the nearest house is not within shouting distance. Their home is beautifully furnished with colonial style throughout. In the dining room are a mahogany table, chairs and sideboard. The table is set with silver and cut glass. There is a delightful drawing room (den), in which there is a small bar, although Frank and Nancy drink little if at all. When we are there – we do.

The kitchen is also an eating area for everyday use. It is modern and so laid out and lavishly equipped to quicken a woman's heart. Every cupboard and the enormous fridge are packed with foods of every description. There is no want in this home.

The bedrooms each contain a four poster bed. Our room had a bathroom and toilet adjoining with colour co-ordinated everything, and thick pile towels of every size.

There is a classical wooden veranda at the back of the house complete with a classical rocking chair. The garage beside the house has a large apartment above it. Behind the garage is a terrace complete with barbecue facilities. Above the front door hangs the American flag. Frank would like to have the Confederate flag there instead – or as well.

Lavish as everything was, the welcome was even more so. Our lifestyles are so different I wonder why we mix so well. I think it helps that Nancy B and I are so much older than they, old enough to be their parents and the grandparents of their children. Nancy A is a charming loving woman and Frank has a sense of humour which is coloured by his language and accent, so typical of the southern states of America which I find fascinating.

Frank has a radiological practice in a purpose built medical centre. The practice is equipped with the latest technology and he provides a diagnostic service for the community of a high standard in keeping with current medical developments. He works single-handed and this has disadvantages. Doctors need to have colleagues with whom to discuss a doubtful or difficult case. Frank has no such colleague. It helps to have colleagues whose company acts as a stimulus and whose conversation can be encouraging on a daily basis. I worry that Frank has to rely so much on himself that there is more strain and anxiety than one would wish. I haven't the necessary grit to work in this way. It would be natural under these circumstances to have periods of doubt and disillusionment. Frank says his most happy times were when he was doing the locum at the Brompton Hospital in London. This doesn't surprise me as there he was surrounded by colleagues of like mind and training who daily are an emotional support. However I'm convinced there are few people who could provide the continuing quality of radiological expertise for the community as Frank does.

On this first visit Frank and Nancy A had a barbecue on the terrace with local friends. Frank did the cooking and the steaks were enormous and succulent. The friends included a few doctors, accountants and lawyers. In modern society doctors need accountants and lawyers, and especially so in America. The conversation that night was lively, witty and with many one-liners at which the Americans are adept. This was our first experience of home life and entertainment in America, so different from our times in city hotels. It was most enjoyable.

Nancy A and Frank are committed Baptists and practise their religion on a daily basis.

Grace is said with every meal, even in restaurants including McDonalds. I admire their strong faith which they extend to others in the community. Nancy A gives time to their church and teaches in the Sunday School. Frank is a respected member of the church and is involved whenever possible in church activities.

We all went to the church on Sunday morning. It is a huge white clapperboard building, set in a large open space with a tall spire dominating the area. The sight of it alone broadcasts an evangelical message. Large cars drove to the massive car park, which was soon full. We walked through the clean, wide, sparkling vestibule into the church with its beautiful wooden pews, large choir stalls and massive organ.

Fortunately Frank had warned us to be early as the church was packed. There was not one empty seat. I thought of our half empty churches in the United Kingdom. The congregation were of all ages, unlike in the United Kingdom where there are few between the ages of seventeen and thirty. There were as many men as women, unlike at home where the women greatly outnumber the men. The atmosphere was one of happiness and enthusiasm, which was reflected in the choir and the singing from the pews. Everyone had dressed for the service; there were no open necked shirts and the ladies wore smart clothes. The preacher was young, large, heavily built and smartly dressed. In the Baptist tradition he wore a collar and tie but no robes. I've now heard him preach a few times since that visit and each sermon was fiery, hard hitting with a clear strong message. In many ways it reminds me of the hell and damnation preaching of a bygone age. There is no room for doubt and this good man is positive about everything. On each occasion I left feeling my doubts would condemn me to damnation. I have so many unanswered questions. However I take consolation from a sermon I heard preached in St Paul's Cathedral in London. The minister, whom I thought highly intelligent said, 'Don't be afraid or worried about your doubts. It's normal to question, and you should, as otherwise you don't think. Think and question and it will help you get it right.'

However I keep searching and my deepest questions remain unanswered. Faith is the opposite to certainty and I yearn for the faith to bring the peace that passes all understanding.

Frank took a holiday from his busy practice to bring us to his condominium by the estuary of the Pungo River. Nancy A and B, Meg, Ross, Frank and I got into the Multiple People Vehicle and set off on the four hour drive. The comfort of the large car made the journey easy. Their large apartment sits in a forest by the river bank.

Sitting on the veranda in the peace and stillness you can hear little but the lapping of the water, as you look over the estuary. You feel a million miles away from the rush and turmoil of towns and cities. Frank has two plots nearby where he plans to build a house. He has a boat in a marina some yards away, where there is also a swimming pool. The pool and shopping facilities are looked after by a young attractive shapely woman whose assets are always on display. She is good at chatting up the men, but Nancy A is always on hand to referee the situation when Frank is the target.

In the forest you can find possum, racoon, wild turkey, deer and even bear.

'Tonight we'll go shining.'

'Frank, what's shining?'

'You'll see. We do this in the car.'

Frank had a powerful light and after dark we drove through the forest. The light attracted the animals and we saw many, including a bear. Mesmerized by the light they just stood and stared, their eyes shining like coloured mirrors.

We slept well that night in a beautiful ensuite bedroom. Of course everything was colour co-ordinated and the towels soft and thick. The apartment had three double sized bedrooms and was airy and light.

The next morning as we sat on the veranda, Frank told me about the Roanoke tribe of Indians who lived in this region until the white man drove them out. I thought we all had a lot to answer for and as we pushed forward our material values others suffered.

As I sat later in the dusk looking across the estuary at the trees lining the river, I could imagine Indian braves coming from behind them to the water edge. I felt compelled to capture the moment. Not being an artist I wrote a poem.

A Tribe in North Carolina

Soft warm air, lapping water,
tall pine trees, white board houses,
the wide Pungo River passing
to the sound in North Carolina.

Looking to the farther shore
longing to see Roanoke
in their hunting land, the silence
holds the ghosts of tribal voices.

Possum, racoon and graceful deer,
shy black bear and pelican
live on the land the braves have left,
driven out by foreign foes.

Slick sailing boats slide past
on tons of dollars.
No wigwams here, no totem poles,
but roller blades and Chevrolets.

A rich marina on the shore,
powered boats, the toys of city folk,
and local shrimp boats with extended arms,
drag and desecrate the river bed.

The new white tribes
with courtesy and charm say 'How y'all?'
but I can hear the crying of the braves,
and as the trees move in the wind,
the wailing of their women.

When we visited Frank and Nancy a year or so later they took us to the State Fair. The fair was big, the hotdogs were big, the drinks were big with enough ice to sink the Titanic. I learnt to say, 'not so much ice please.' There was food everywhere, baked, barbecued and roasted. There were country crafts of every description and Nancy B bought a nice silver ring. We saw fewer animals than at home. Everything was on such a grand scale that I wondered why Frank and Nancy A loved our Guildford County Show so much. Perhaps being smaller it was more intimate and the show jumping certainly had a particularly English flavour to it. The vintage cars were also typically British.

For the first time Nancy B and I saw State Troopers at close quarters. They are a police force but more like a trained army. I've never seen in any of my travels a smarter looking body of men and women. I'm told, and believe it, that their efficiency matches their appearance. They wear stiff Baden-Powell hats, grey shirts crisply starched and ironed in creases, grey trousers with a charcoal side stripe and black shoes polished to perfection. Their trouser creases would cut your arm as their holstered side guns would end your life. The men were all clean shaved and short haired. Frank has great admiration and respect for them. 'They're all college graduates and, I tell you, you don't mess with these boys.'

As the fair closed for the evening there was a firework display. It was such a mixture of noise and colour that I thought it could be seen and heard in London, and it went on and on, getting bigger and better. Nancy B, who loves fireworks more than I, was mesmerized.

The next day we set off for the Blue Ridge mountains. The highways were long, large and wide. We passed through one-street linear towns with gas stations, car lots, cafes of many types and hoardings advertising all the material wealth of the land including food, furniture and female finery. These linear towns are not a pretty sight, but the scene changed when we reached the mountain range. Trees of every variety covered the slopes and peaks, producing a kaleidoscope of colour beyond imagination. Only the human eye could capture the beauty, which is beyond the ability of a camera and is a challenge to the most skilled artists. There is no canvas that could hold the gold, copper, rust, dark and olive green, orange and yellow that nature blended into one. If there is a heaven this was it and if there is a God this is his work. All lay within a blue haze which later in the setting sun became purple. It was as if the colours had a liquid quality constantly changing and flowing. Looking up, the sky was a cloudless blue, and looking down from the peaks you saw a multicoloured carpet. We drove to a height over one mile high and feasted on this scene to the bursting of our senses. It was a sacrilege to speak.

We were heading for Cherokee country, part of the reason for the trip. We stayed overnight in Waynesville, in the Smoky Mountain Inn. The next morning we drove to the Cherokee village. Nancy B and I had never seen American Indians. Unlike the popular image of Indians the Cherokee don't wear the feather headdress or the leather clothes.

These are a mountain tribe that survived on farming. Their dark eyed, dark haired and dark skinned Mongolian features spoke of their origin more than their checked shirts and trousers. For the tourist trade however some had worn the feathers and the leather. In the 1880s fifty thousand of this tribe were resettled by the government of the day and their reluctant journey was known as the Trail of Tears. Five thousand died on that trek. Some refused to go and hid in mountain caves. Their descendants lived in this village and now survived mainly by tourism.

We had a guided tour and learnt of their customs and crafts. They were converted to Christianity by the white man, who also brought aggression and disease. They were scourged by smallpox. An intelligent tribe, they were the first to have an alphabet. The guided tour was interesting and their crafts were many including excellent pottery, but I was sad at the sight of this native tribe, whose dignity was reduced, living as a second class people in their own land, on a reservation with restrictions imposed by the dominant white race.

We returned the next day to Fuquay-Varina, looking forward to attending our first ever American college football game. This was between Clemson University where Frank graduated and the University of North Carolina, where his friend Brent Barringer, an attorney, graduated. Their friendly rivalry generated an amusing banter. Kick off time was 5.45 p.m., and was preceded by the spectators having picnics from the backs of their large vehicles, mostly four wheel drives. The Americans call this 'tail gating'. The food characteristically was lavish. Lager was drunk instead of wine. We feasted like medieval barons on the best of meats, vegetables and breads of indescribable varieties, laid out on large portable tables.

There was no poverty around these fields!

Well satisfied, warm and comfortable we took our seats in the stadium. It was enormous. Mini skirted cheer leaders danced and acrobated on the side lines. Large brass bands for each team played and paraded on the field, marching back and forward in ever changing patterns, each band made up of students in the university, for which they wore the colours. The air of carnival was everywhere.

Then a voice came from the loudspeaker announcing that a minute's silence would be taken in honour of the seventeen naval men and women killed by a terrorist bomb in Aden. Fifty thousand people stood. The silence was sudden and spectacular.

Around me I saw some women wipe their tears. The atmosphere was solemn and emotional. It was to get more so, as these fifty thousand sang the Star Spangled Banner. I too felt a tear, identifying totally with the sentiment they expressed. I said to Nancy B, 'It's this emotion and this togetherness that keeps this vast and varied country united.' I wondered if these qualities were still alive in the United Kingdom. I so much want them to be so.

When the game began the mood changed. Brent was jumping, shouting, swearing, clapping, elated and despondent in turns. It was almost hysterical. It was hysterical. To my surprise Frank was quiet and composed. The manoeuvres on the field seemed like a physical form of chess, played at high speed but with frequent intervals. There was more subtlety in the moves than the physical activity displayed. When the player crosses the opponents' goal line carrying the ball it is called a 'touch down', and is a score. However unlike rugby, the player doesn't have to touch the ball on the ground – strange. At this game, one 'touch down' was achieved by the player somersaulting over the battle-locked warriors on the line. I've never seen such a thing and wondered why we don't try that when the scrum is on the opponents' line in rugby. There is much tackling in American football and the game is indeed very physical as players are impeded when not carrying the ball. Each tackle and move was greeted by shouts of triumph or yells of woe from the crowd, all in high spirits and fun. There was none of the aggressive and loutish behaviour that blights the national game of football in the United Kingdom and Europe. As the crowd left the stadium friends and foes greeted each other with smiles and good humour. Sport should always be like this. I'm aware that this was a University game and in the UK rugby matches have the same atmosphere, but Frank confirms that the national games of football in America are not associated with rowdy and destructive behaviour.

A day later we were off again to the condominium by the Pungo River. As we sat on the veranda I wanted to write something about our trip. Frank said, 'Ah think ah will try to write somethin'. Ah's got an idee from my past.'

He wrote a story as we sat there and read it to me. It was about a day in a boat out shooting and the characters were a man and a young boy. It was clear that this was Frank and his father on Frank's first hunting trip. I was immediately captivated by the writing. I admit it took me by surprise and I hadn't expected Frank to have this skill. As he read, this tough, rugged, swearing and macho man – wept. I warmed to Frank, more complex than I knew, and felt my tears just below the surface.

The story was moving and flowed effortlessly. It was pure Hemingway. I thought of my struggles with composition and felt humble as Frank wrote this vivid tale that illustrated genuine talent.

'Frank, you have a gift. You must write more.'

I haven't seen another story yet but hope I will. While Frank wrote I composed a poem, but it is a poor effort compared to Frank's. It does express however the trip to the Indian tribe.

The Cherokee

Drive south on Interstate 40
then North Carolina 181
along Blue Ridge Parkway
till the setting of the sun.

The Blue Ridge mountains magic
beauty seldom seen,
yellow, gold and russet brown,
copper and olive green.

To the home of the Cherokee Indians
centuries gone by,
a noble race of farming folk
content where their mountains lie.

Then came the warring white man,
gunpowder and disease,
who drove them from their homeland
while speaking still of peace.

Fifty thousand were moved out
along the Trail of Tears,
five thousand died along the way
with horrors each one fears.

But some remained in hiding
in the mountain caves
separated from their kinfolk
and their broken Indian braves.

Today in the reservation
we see this Indian tribe
acting for the tourists
bereft of their ancient pride.

We have destroyed a people,
denied them their given land
to impose a different life style
not worth a grain of sand.

Chapter 19

Retirement

As I moved toward sixty five years of age, the age of compulsory retirement for consultants in the National Health Service, I became increasingly anxious. Friends and colleagues spoke to Nancy but only to pose the question, 'My God, what are you going to do with Oscar when he retires?' I detected that Nancy too was worried.

As the time approached, 1992 was the relevant date, I thought of many ways to spend my time, but never reached a satisfactory decision. My life in medicine had been so full, my life at home had been so happy. The girls had moved out to successful careers and started families themselves. How would I fill my time? I loved teaching medicine. I would miss this and I would miss the students. Some colleagues did locums. I would hate to do that. I had no hobbies – another mistake. Could I carry on with my medico-legal work? Yes, but that didn't provide the busy life I needed, and I must be careful not to carry on too long. I did continue on the Cases Committee of the Medical Protection Society and was a member of the President's Advisory Board until I was seventy two, but stopped being an expert medical witness before I lost my credibility.

I remembered Dr Harold Edwards, consultant neurologist and Past Dean of St Mary's Hospital Medical School, one night at our dining table in a very bad mood. A dinner guest said, 'Harold, what's wrong with you tonight? You're in very bad form.'

'I'll tell you what's wrong,' he replied.

'All my life I've been achieving in one way or another, often in small ways but others significant, but achieving nonetheless. Since retirement I've achieved nothing.'

Suddenly I realized that what drove me and my colleagues in medicine was to achieve. We needed to make a contribution to life.

Could I continue to lecture? Surprisingly, invitations to lecture continued to come and I spoke often on medical topics, but increasingly on medico-legal subjects, especially informed consent which was very topical in the 1990s. To my surprise and delight I continued to get invitations to give after dinner speeches. These were many and often people would say ' Oscar, you seem to be as busy as ever.'

'Don't you believe it. You must have no idea how busy my life was and this is nothing like it.'

I missed being President of the College. There is nothing as past as a past President, I had no further input into the College and think it a mistake that the College doesn't use its Past Officers enough. It would be a contribution even to chair some scientific meetings and we hadn't lost the ability to introduce speakers.

Why had I given up golf? I gave up many years ago to free the weekends and give time to my children. There was another reason however – I played golf very badly and this frustrated me. It would be the same if I started again. The last thing I needed was frustration.

Soon my restlessness increased. Should I move house? Perhaps I should move to the country. The one hobby I did enjoy in the past was horse riding. I had stopped after an abdominal operation for my perforated gall bladder in 1985. I could start riding again. Yes, that was possible. I could buy a house in the country with stabling and keep a horse. That would occupy me. I thought about this for a long time and the appeal of it grew. In the mornings when I woke up my thoughts turned with pleasure to the stable with its mixture of smells. I always loved the smell of manure. It's fresh and brings up memories of my youth, holidays in the country, my grandparents' stables and the pleasures of riding good horses. I love the smell of leather and indeed the touch of it. Saddling a horse is exciting in itself. What a good idea. I would take part in the local shows. I would play a part in village life.

I would change church and maybe get on the Parish Council. Yes, I could see a whole new life open up for me. I would need more county clothes instead of city suits. My riding boots would still fit me. I should make this change before it's too late. I will talk to Nancy about it.

Nancy listened to my suggestions with a face that registered increasing horror.

'You would have to "muck out" the stable, feed and groom the horse yourself, day in and day out in all weathers. You couldn't leave the house and the horse unattended for any time. What would you do in the winter? What would you do in the country when not on the horse? You do know you love shopping. You do know you love the buzz of London. You still meet your colleagues in the Royal Society of

Medicine. You know it is in 1 Wimpole Street. You enjoy having tea, lunch or dinner there. We have our Freedom Passes – free travel in London on trains and buses. You lose that in the country. You love the theatre and the Festival Hall. You are a town man for goodness sake. Think again.'

What she said was true. I did love shopping especially in Fortnum and Mason's and Harrods. I loved Jermyn Street. I dallied happily in John Lewis in Oxford Street and sauntered through the back door to Cavendish Square and on to the RSM in Wimpole Street. I loved having coffee in Chelsea watching the world go by, and what a varied world! The girls are getting younger and prettier as I grow older but watching them keeps my mind younger. Even such frustration is stimulating.

In retirement I had also found the delights of the Royal Academy. It was in Piccadilly! My daughter Louise had given me membership each year as a birthday present. I had always loved music and Nancy and I went to the Festival Hall, often with Alistair and Grethe Dykes. Alistair, now retired, had been the minister of the church we attended, St Andrews Presbyterian, Cheam. We loved going to the theatre in Richmond, often with Robert and Gertie Steiner.

I was chastened by Nancy's opinion and yet knowing in my heart she was right, tried to resist it. I cannot ignore Nancy's opinion on matters such as this and am convinced she knows what is best for everyday living. I gently ran her thoughts through my mind for some time and then said, 'Darling, I don't think it would be a good idea to move to the country. After all we can get to the country very easily from Cheam and even to the seaside. Do you know, I think I'm a town man.'

'Oscar, I think you're right.'

Although we were settling into a retired pattern it was taking some time and there was still no achievement. I wasn't satisfied. Nancy and I attend church regularly and I was an ordained Elder in the Presbyterian Church which now was called the United Reformed Church. I had heard many sermons on the use of whatever talents we might have and how we should serve our fellow man. I thought with my experience of lecturing and teaching I might have some part to play in the life of the church. The time might be right for me to become a lay preacher. Yes, this could be a life of achievement. I got quite excited about this possibility and still find it exciting.

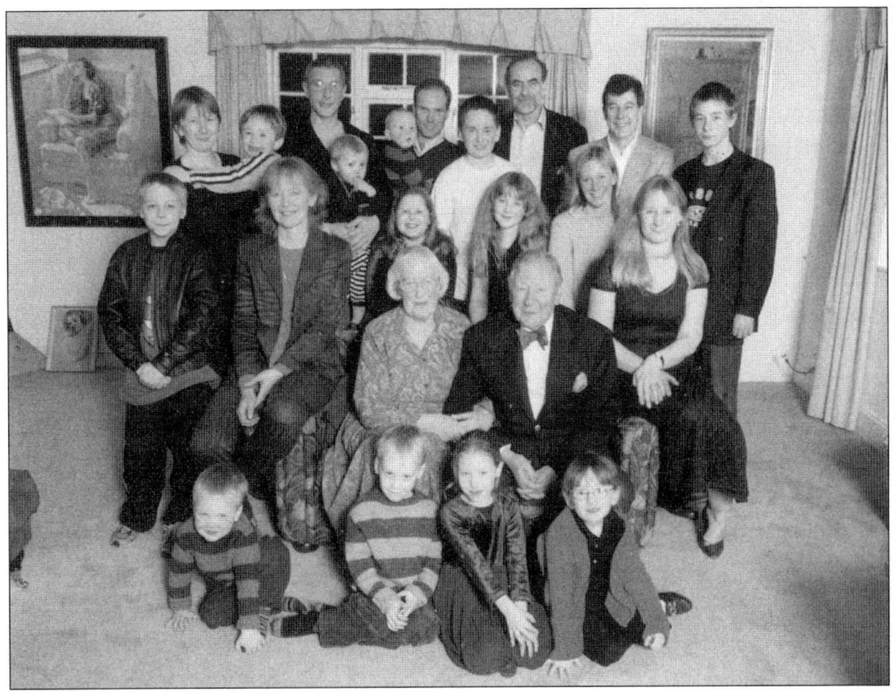

The author and Nancy with daughters, sons-in-law and grandchildren

But I have to look deeply into my motives. Am I attracted to preaching just to occupy my time? Do I wish to preach just to occupy centre stage? I have a great love of centre stage! What about my suitability to preach? Before applying for acceptance or for any teaching course I needed to answer these questions. My youngest daughter, Sheena, married to Alistair Tresidder, Vicar of St Luke's Church, Hampstead, knows my mind well and says I would never be accepted. I fear she is right. My Christianity is unorthodox. My doubts are strong and my faith is weak. I have my own interpretation of biblical events. Was it leprosy that was healed or was it psoriasis? Was it a virgin birth or did virgin just mean 'a young girl'? Many such questions plague me. Nonetheless I cannot find a better solution to the good life for me than following Christian teaching and for me life without Jesus Christ seems shallow, but I hesitate to convert others. Can we offer anything better than the Jewish faith, or the Hindu and Moslem religions? Many of my closest and dearest friends in medicine are atheists and their contribution to their fellow man is an example to follow. I wonder if it matters, as it says in John, Chapter 15, verse 16, 'It is not that you chose me, but

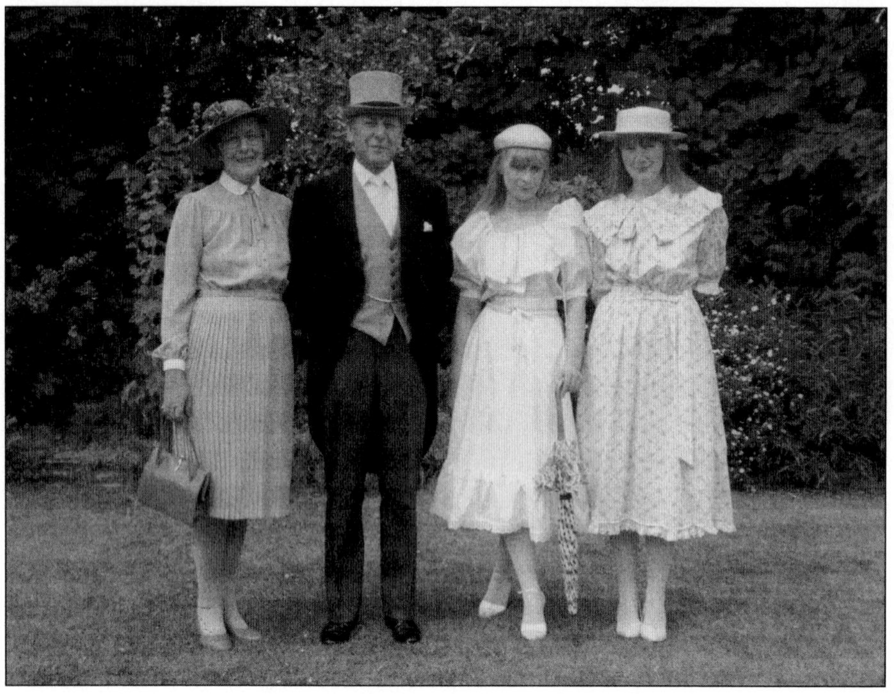

Dressed for the Buckingham Palace Garden Party. Left to right Nancy, author, Louise and Finella.

that I chose you'. I am forced to the conclusion that it would be almost profane for me to preach from the pulpit, but deeply regret it may be so.

When visiting the College I saw the portraits of past Presidents on the wall. I thought it would be a good idea to write their history. I interviewed those still alive and did some superficial research. I wrote a sample chapter. It was significantly bad without me knowing it at the time. I had an opinion from the editor in the Royal Society of Medicine at the time, Howard Croft. When I told him I didn't write well he smiled at my modesty and said he would let me know. He sent me a letter which said, 'You are right'. I decided to enrol in a Creative Writing class in the Sutton College of Liberal Arts (SCOLA). This opened up a new world to me and a new chapter in my life. After some time I began writing essays. During this time I realized that a book on the Past Presidents would be boring. At least I couldn't make it interesting without details of their personalities and anecdotes about their lives and perhaps I should postpone this for the time being. I should try something easier. Many of the essays I had written were about my life as a child which the tutor had suggested. I realized I could attempt an autobiography. With considerable effort I managed to write and publish *A Life in Medicine*, with the help and encouragement of Ian and Marjory Chapman, friends from church and themselves professional editors and publishers of distinction. The thrill of writing this book was fantastic and at last I was achieving. Nancy during these years had joined an art class in SCOLA and loves painting which she does with increasing skill. My retirement was becoming more interesting.

My friend John Laws and his wife Diana, (née Brinkley), a clinical oncologist, belonged to the Harveian Society of London and proposed me for membership. The Harveian is a medical society founded to honour William Harvey who, in 1628, was the first doctor to describe the circulation of the blood correctly. The Society meets monthly in Lettsom House, Chandos Street, London. It was founded in 1831 'for the purpose of discussing medical, surgical and philosophical subjects, connected with medical subjects'. Nancy comes to these meetings as my guest, although she is eligible for membership, and following a buffet supper a lecture is delivered by an invited speaker. Here I keep in touch, meet old colleagues and foster new ones. Some time after joining I was elected to Council. Later I was appointed Junior Secretary and then Senior Secretary. In the year 2001, I was appointed President-Elect. That year I chose the speakers for my year as President in 2002. As President I chaired Council and the monthly meetings of members. It was a full year and I will deal with some aspects of it later.

All in all retirement is a pleasure, with enough achievement to satisfy me, even though I still miss the cut and thrust of hospital practice.

Nancy and I travel for pleasure now and not just to give lectures. Trips to France are easy and enjoyable. I like walking and often drive to Ham through Richmond Park to walk by the Thames. Nancy has developed some arthritis in her knees and cannot walk far with me, so sits and paints by the river. We bought a beach hut in Goring-on-Sea. We can drive there in just over an hour from Cheam. We have a small gas burner in the hut and it is a joy to have bacon and eggs on the beach.

We enjoy giving dinner or lunch parties at home and this keeps us in contact with medical colleagues and local friends. There is time for this now.

Recently we became members of the Medical Society of London which meets twice monthly, also in Lettsom House. The format is the same as the Harveian Society of London.

I've been retired for just over ten years now and life is full. It took time to settle, and I still need to achieve. This book is part of this need and when I finish it I will need to search again. As I write this sentence I'm aware I need to be fit above all else, to do anything. I worry about Nancy's health and mine. I've told many patients in my time that I'm a professional hypochondriac, but am aware that as age advances illness becomes more and more possible. There is no prize greater than good health.

A large part of my life rests in my four daughters, Siobhan, Louise, Finella and Sheena. I'm proud of each and the fathers of my twelve grandchildren. Each of my daughters made good choices in their men and each is successful. Above all other considerations, this enlarged family holds pride of place. I thank God for them.

Chapter 20

An Ecumenical Service

When I began my medical studies two years were spent on the dissection of the human body. This was to teach the student the details of anatomy, muscle by muscle, nerve by nerve, artery by artery, vein by vein and organ by organ. It was not a hurried study but learnt piece by piece, day by day. The dissection was aided by complex anatomical texts and dissecting manuals. Though not the purpose of the work, we learnt also the use of the scalpel.

We were so young and ignorant of medicine, that the importance of the study of anatomy partly escaped us. We did our dissection and our reading to pass on to the next stage in our course. To many it was tedious. Much later in our medical careers the inestimable value of anatomical study became apparent. Nonetheless countless hours were spent in the dissecting room.

In my memory I see a strangely Victorian setting, with lines of tables, on which lay the naked bodies, taken each morning from a formalin bath. Surprisingly we were unaffected by what I now see as a gruesome image. For some reason we didn't associate these bodies with the living, or weren't affected by who they had been or what lives they had led. Today I would be unable to be so detached. On reflection our lack of emotion was a protection, without which we would have been unsettled. We sat around each table in small groups, feeling and dissecting while inhaling the pungent smell of formalin.

Our Professor of Anatomy was Professor Evatt, a very small, bald, moustached man who had been a Colonel in the Royal Army Medical Corps. He was kind, conscientious, elderly and deaf. He lectured but was seldom seen in the dissecting room. At each table was an anatomy demonstrator, either a lecturer in the department, or a surgeon who volunteered to teach. The surgeons were the most popular teachers, as they related the anatomy to surgical practice and emphasized the application of anatomy to particular operations. Others taught anatomy as a science in itself, but medical students didn't think of it as such. Senior medical students were sometimes chosen as demonstrators and I was fortunate to be one in my clinical years. This was my first introduction to teaching in medicine.

A remarkable character, Tom Gary, taught anatomy at the Royal College of Surgeons in Ireland. Not medically qualified, he was a pure anatomist. It was acknowledged by students and senior medical men that nobody knew the anatomy of the human body better than Tom Gary. Tom would introduce himself with the words,

'In darkest Africa where they have never heard of Jesus Christ, Tom Gary is a household name.

Not only was Tom a college character, he was known throughout the medical profession in Ireland. He was a familiar figure in Dublin, small with an elfin face and mischievous eyes, a cigarette always dangling from his lips, wearing a black homburg and a black coat green and shining with age. He taught anatomy in a sonorous Shakespearian voice, detailing the subject with lyrical phrases. With little prior knowledge he was difficult to follow, but with a basic understanding his teaching became dazzling. He lived in York Street, beside the Royal College of Surgeons, where he kept a body on which he gave private tutorials. These were invaluable for those studying for the Part 1 of the Fellowship of the Royal College of Surgeons, when anatomical knowledge would be severely tested. I attended these tutorials and was amazed to find his rooms lined and partitioned by columns of books and his bed in a room only separated from the dissecting table and the body by books. Tom wasn't married and that was fortunate. He was respected by students as a senior academic and even more so by countless Dublin surgeons.

When we studied anatomy in the 1940s the details of cross-sectional anatomy were not stressed. Cross-sectional anatomy is the study of the body, seen as though looking into the body, at right angles to the long axis, at varying levels. In those days it had a limited application and little did we know how important it was to become three decades later. With the invention of Computed Tomography (CT scanning) and Magnetic Resonance Imaging (MRI) the living body is seen in cross section at varying levels. Cross sectional anatomy has taken on great importance. Less time is now spent by students on cadaver dissection. This is a loss and reflects on the student's basic knowledge, about which I hear complaints from my colleagues. Cadaver dissection remains an essential, especially for surgeons. For this experience it is necessary to have bodies donated to medical schools and postgraduate medical colleges. Fortunately donors still exist and this act on the part of the donor is a great sacrifice. Relatives are to some extent denied a public farewell that marks the end of the life of their loved one.

I was unaware until some years ago that a church service is held annually in London to give thanks for the bodies that have been donated during the year. Relatives are invited and the service is attended by members of London University and the clergy of different denominations. It is truly ecumenical. I learnt about this event wheh I was invited to give the address at the service to be held on Friday, 20 May 1994, in the University Church of Christ the King, Gordon Square, London. I had been retired two years.

The church is large and it was packed with relatives, and I was delighted to see many medical students present. It was a solemn and dignified occasion. The university members wore academic dress and the clergy were suitably robed. The organist was Mr Simon Over and the choir was made up of the University of London Church Choir and the St Mary's Hospital Medical School Choir.

I gave the following address:

Lord, may the thoughts of my mind and the words of my mouth be acceptable in your sight.

We are here today to give thanks for all those men and women who donated their bodies for medical and dental education and research.

The text of my address is Hebrews, Chapter 13 Verse 16, 'And do not forget to do good and to share with others, for with such sacrifices God is pleased.'

George Eliot wrote,
'For the growing good of the world is partly dependent on unhistoric acts; and that things are not so ill with you and me as they might have been, is half owing to the number who lived faithfully a hidden life and rest in unvisited tombs.'

The quality of medicine that we practise today is due to a slow gradual development since the years before Christ, but the advances in the last few decades have surpassed imagination. Biochemical tests have reached a surprising sophistication and represent an exact science as never before. Genetics provide a window into congenital disease and may prove the key for the prevention of some intolerable disorders and perhaps even a route to the defeat of cancer. In my own field, isotope imaging, ultrasound, CT scanning and Magnetic Resonance have enabled precise diagnoses in all areas of the body. The brain, heart, blood vessels and abdominal organs have never been visualized so clearly in the living patient. In recent years organ movement and the circulation have been seen in real time, that is to say, in motion in fractions of seconds. Clinical radiology has made dramatic contributions to surgery and clinical radiologists dilate diseased arteries, drain abscess cavities, perform diagnostic aspirations and bypass procedures in the biliary tract and elsewhere to give quantity and quality of life. Surgical techniques have surpassed expectation in organ transplantation, including heart, lung, liver and kidney organs singly or in multiples. Joint surgery and prosthetic surgery enable the crippled to walk and advances in brain and eye surgery give sight to the blind and power to the weak.

Endocrine diseases have been controlled by physicians and surgeons. Diptheria, smallpox, plague, malaria, tuberculosis and other infections can be treated and eliminated. The treatment of cancer by radiotherapy, cytotoxic drugs or combinations of both is gradually moving to the final defeat of this scourge of the human race. How did we ever reach this advanced stage?

It isn't possible in one address to tell the full story of medical achievement, but some salient facts can be covered. Medical achievement begins in the medical school where the first steps in medical education begin. I am privileged to lecture to medical students and in common with many other medical teachers I have emphasized that unless the basic anatomy of the human body is thoroughly learnt and understood, not only will the knowledge of medicine be incomplete but progress and discovery could well be inhibited or even halted.

The Christian Church from its earliest times has felt a duty to nurture the sick and feed the poor. The church founded the first hospitals and one of these early churches still stands on the island of Rhodes, established during the crusades by the Knights of St John. Even thought the church encouraged these caring and nursing activities, it had serious objections to the dissection of the human body, and it cannot be denied that this impeded the progress of medical knowledge at that time. Over the years ecclesiastical thinking was to modify and today a close bond exists between the teachings of the church and the practice of medicine. Of course the church still feels obliged to voice its opinion when in some areas of medicine ethics and morals need to be considered. What is scientifically possible is not always morally acceptable. The need for laws in medicine goes back to Hammurabi, one of the earliest kings of Babylon, who drew up laws for medical practice about 1948 years BC.

Because of the attitude to human dissection, anatomy didn't progress for centuries, but in 1543 with the publication of Fabrica Humani Corporis, Andreas Vesalius initiated an immense and spectacular change. He challenged the existing authorities on anatomical science based on earlier written observations, and described the structure of the human body such as he found it by dissection, i.e. by looking at things as they were. It is interesting that one of the monks in charge of the hospital in Venice where Vesalius worked was Ignatius Loyola who formed the Order of Jesuits for the spiritual welfare of mankind. Vesalius by teaching what he himself had seen, and what he could make his students see, brought into anatomy a new heart and intelligence. This was the beginning of modern anatomy and physiology. So, great advances followed. It was from dissection that knowledge of the brain, the nerves and their pathways, joints and tendons, the structure of the heart, abdominal organs, vascular pathways and the lymphatic system was obtained.

Knowledge was added piecemeal, bit by bit and man by man.

I quote, 'the greatness of all men is built partly on the worth of those who have gone before.'

So Harvey, born in Folkestone in 1578 appointed physician to St Bartholomew's Hospital in 1609 at the age of thirty one, with his great illustration of the circulation of the blood in 1628, did for physiology what Vesalius had done for anatomy. It is said that Harvey's work was the direct outcome of the teaching of Vesalius.

In 1590 the brothers Hans and Zacharius Janssen in Holland invented the microscope, later perfected by Cornelius Drebbel. So anatomical dissection moved to the description of elemental structure. Gross anatomy had led to microscopic anatomy which in turn led to physiological advances.

Great anatomical names of the times were Malpighi of Bologna, Stensen of Denmark, Hooke of London, Swammerdam of Amsterdam and van Leevenhoek of Delft. Willis, an Englishman, in 1664 described features of the cerebral circulation which still bear his name.

All was not easy however. Alexander Munro (1697–1767) was appointed Professor of Anatomy in Edinburgh at the age of twenty two. He found it necessary to seek sanctuary within the university in 1725 because of a public demonstration against body snatching. In 1824 Robert Knox was the most popular anatomist in Edinburgh, a brilliant orator and inspiring teacher. At the height of his career, Burke and Hare sold him a body for £7.10s and so were encouraged to commit a series of murders, the last of whose body was found in the rooms of Robert Knox.

Knox fell into disfavour although totally innocent of any fault. Although he recovered from this, he gradually lost his power and position. There are many stories of the difficulties of performing anatomical dissections. They illustrate that anatomical knowledge was not achieved by chance or with comfort, but by determination, dedication, commitment and sacrifice.

Winston Churchill said in 1944 when addressing the Royal College of Physicians, 'the longer you can look back, the further you can look forward.' Our knowledge of anatomy goes back a long way and it leads to looking forward to what we can and will do. On the bricks of basic dissection we build the future doctors and those that will advance the comfort and well-being of human life.

When I was thinking of this address I spoke to Professor Harold Ellis, a celebrated surgeon and teacher of anatomy, and Professor Norman Browse, President of the Royal College of Surgeons about the importance of anatomy and dissection of the human body. They both paid tribute to the availability of dissection by which means not only did the student learn anatomy, but also developed a sense of touch and feel that helped to develop an enormous respect for the body and its structure, and consequently the way it should be handled. This also helped the student develop a psychological approach to the patient. For the training of doctors and surgeons models are not good enough, and those that bequest their bodies to anatomy schools do the public an enormous service. The knowledge gained leads to developments in all branches of medicine and surgery.

Today we give thanks to all those who by donating their bodies have contributed so much to these advances. Their sacrifice places a solemn burden on all members of the medical profession, so to deport themselves that their work, commitment and compassion pay tribute to these honourable men and women.

I end as I began,

'For the growing good of the world is partly dependent on unhistoric acts; and that things are not so ill with you and me as they might have been, is half owing to the number who lived faithfully a hidden life and rest in unvisited tombs.'

May the grace of God remain with them forever.

Amen.

CHAPTER 21

The Harveian Society of London

IN RETIREMENT I BECAME a member of the Harveian Society of London founded in 1831. I regret I didn't belong earlier in my career, but life was busy and I gave a tutorial to medical postgraduates, trainees in clinical radiology, on Wednesday evenings, the evening the Harveian Society met. Now I look forward to every meeting. I enjoy the buffet supper, the wine and especially the company. Here I also meet old colleagues and make new ones. The lectures are invariably excellent and apart from medical topics include the arts, painting, travel, history and on one recent occasion tapestry. A presidential lecture some years ago was on archaeology.

William Harvey was born in Folkestone on 1st April 1578, during the reign of Elizabeth I and in the year of the Spanish Armada. He was the eldest son of Thomas Harvey, a prosperous Kentish yeoman. Thomas Harvey introduced a postal service to Kent and in 1586 was elected mayor of Folkestone. When aged 10 in 1588 William entered King's School, Canterbury. He won the Matthew Parker scholarship, when aged 15 and entered Caius College Cambridge, where he spent three years studying classics, philosophy and physics. He took his BA degree in 1597. John Caius had given permission in his statutes for medical study in one of four universities, Padua, Verona, Montpelier or Paris. Like Caius, Harvey chose Padua, the most renowned university for medical study at the time. He left for Padua in October 1599. On arriving at Dover to take the boat to Calais, the harbour captain put him in jail. The boat sank during a storm, with the loss of many of Harvey's friends. The captain said he had a dream the night before with the request to stop Harvey. (This is a strange story but no other details are available to me. I wonder on what charge Harvey was placed in jail.)

He arrived in Padua in January 1600, and studied under Hieronymous Fabricius ab Aquapendente, the great anatomist. The work of Fabricius on the valves of the veins played a significant role in Harvey's thinking about the circulation of the blood. Harvey's work on embryology began in Padua under the influence of Fabricius. In 1602

Harvey received his doctorate with a 'licence to practise and to teach arts and medicine in every land and seat of learning'.

He returned to England the same year and was granted Licentiate of the College of Physicians. In 1604 he became a Member of the College of Physicians and in that year married Elizabeth Brown, whose father was physician to Elizabeth I and later James I. William and Elizabeth had no children.

In 1607 Harvey was elected a Fellow of the College and two years later, in 1609 was appointed physician to St Bartholomew's Hospital. In 1618 he became Physician Extraordinary to James I.

It was in 1628 that Harvey rocked the medical profession with his publication De Motu Cordis (on the movement of the heart), which described correctly for the first time, the circulation of the blood. His description overturned the writings of Galen and the current beliefs, causing many of his colleagues to believe him misguided. However Harvey's description of the circulation of the blood began the development of modern cardiology and takes its place as one of the most momentous steps in medical history. In 1630 Harvey was made Physician Ordinary to Charles I, who took a keen interest in his work. They became close friends. A renowned painting is one of Harvey demonstrating the heart to Charles. During the Civil War, Harvey attended the King at the Battle of Edgehill. He retreated with Charles to Oxford, where he spent four years and in 1645 was elected Warden of Merton College, Oxford. It isn't surprising that Harvey was elected President of the Royal College of Physicians in 1654, but it is disappointing he declined this honour on account of ill health. He died in his eightieth year on 3rd June 1657, and is buried in Hempstead in Essex, where his family owned land.

Professor Gaetano Thiene of Padua University visited the Harveian Society of London in the year 2000 with the intention of arranging a joint celebration of the 400th anniversary of Harvey's graduation in Padua which was to fall in the year 2002. In 2001 he contacted the Royal College of Physicians to interest them in the celebration, and as a result a joint planning committee of the Royal College of Physicians, the Harveian Society of London and the University of Padua was formed. This was under the chairmanship of Dr Allan Bennett, Treasurer of the Royal College of Physicians. It was decided to hold two symposia, the first to take place in Padua in April 2002 and the second in London in June 2002. It was my good fortune to be President of the Harveian Society of London that year. Each year the Harveian Society and the Medical Society of London have a joint summer trip and in the year 2002 our visit to the celebration in Padua would make an excellent venture. So the invitation to Padua included the Fellows of the Royal College of Physicians, the Harveian Society of London and the Medical Society of London.

We landed at Marco Polo Airport in Venice on Wednesday, 24th April and immediately felt the warmth of Italy. A representative from Focus Tours met us and led us to a waiting coach and reminiscent of our schooldays counted us in. We were almost all retired and enjoyed being cared for in this way. It was comfortable to sit back in a large seat, relaxed and with friends. The coach was full of holiday smiles and chatter.

We sped along the motorway to Padua, past flat countryside, with acres of sparsely cultivated land surrounding poorly decorated farm-houses. There was no hint of wealth in these dwellings and this was an Italy not advertised in tourist brochures. But we could see the mountains in the distance, snow capped and beautiful. We were all well travelled and knew the Italy of sun and song and architectural splendour. Nancy and I, with many of our colleagues, stayed in the Plaza Hotel in Padua. The hotel, with an international flavour, was inviting and the desk clerks, dressed like city executives, spoke perfect English. As always I wished I could speak the language of the country, but even my French is answered with laughter, and I have no Italian whatever.

I was happy to have landed safely and to be there, but now I had to face my fear of lifts. I've been stuck in lifts too many times and now I panic at the sight of one, but Nancy holds my hand and chats me up and down. I walk when possible, but modern hotels often only have emergency stairs. I never go into a lift alone. My pulse has quickened even writing this. Why does it take forever for the doors to open? I am cursed with a vivid imagination. I long for a placid temperament, but advancing years have brought no solace. We reached our room on the third floor. As always on opening the door I said, 'Me first for the toilet'. The room was pleasant but had twin beds although we asked for a double. A sculptured plaque above the bed of a naked shapely woman admiring flowers seemed appropriate and added a touch of Italy to the room. This aura was challenged by the contemporary television set. We didn't use it despite the advertisement on top for erotic movies. We had space and a functional bathroom with plenty of clean towels, soap and a shower.

A formal dinner was planned for 8.00 p.m., so what we needed was a drink and a rest.

'Nancy where is the gin? Have you got your whisky?' We always bring our own. We find it ridiculous to pay so much in hotels for a whisky which only covers the bottom of the glass or a gin which is mostly tonic water.

Dinner was hosted by the Rotary Club of Padua, and they entertained us and our colleagues from the University of Padua. Professor Thiene from the University had organized all the Italian celebrations. To my surprise he began the speeches before the meal. Sir George Alberti, President of the Royal College of Physicians, replied followed by me as President of the Harveian Society of London. The food was good, even the pasta, but the wine was even better. Having made my speech, I could drink the wine without restraint. 'Sure wasn't our bedroom only one floor up from the dining room?'

The lectures began the next day and the symposium was 'Recent Advances in Cardiovascular Medicine'. It was difficult to enter the world of science and scholarship; retirement and the relaxed atmosphere of our trip fought against it.

Many of the lectures were based on laboratory research and many facts had yet to be proved. The visiting audience were mostly clinically based doctors. The lecturers however were international giants in their field.

The University and the lecture theatre had a medieval grandeur that contrasted with the technology of the presentations. I wondered if the ghost of Harvey was in the room, marvelling at the power point slickness of each lecturer's performance.

There are moments in life and images that hit the mind like the explosion of the atom; such a moment and such an image struck when I saw the Anatomy Theatre in Padua.

This theatre was inaugurated on 16th January 1594. Harvey arrived in Padua in 1600 and was taught in this very theatre. It is an impressive beautifully carved wooden structure consisting of circled tiers rising to the roof and holding two hundred students. The central dissecting table on the floor can be seen from every place.

It was conceived and paid for by Fabicius ab Aquapendente, and is the oldest permanent anatomy theatre still in existence today. The design is attributed to Paolo Sarpi (1552–1623). The dissecting table can be turned over hiding the corpse, and revealing an animal. It was said this was to offer comparative anatomy. It the sixteenth and seventeenth centuries music was often played in the Anatomy Theatre, both to keep the students calm while they waited for the teacher and also to produce a relaxed atmosphere.

The official dinner of the symposium was held that evening, Thursday 25th April, a fine occasion. The speeches were held at the coffee stage and again Sir George, Gaetano Thiene and I spoke.

Following a morning of lectures on Friday, we were free to explore Padua. We sauntered wide eyed with pleasure through clean and bright streets, full of restaurants, sophisticated boutiques and pillared walkways. A guided tour included a visit to Battistero del Duomo, the bishop's seat. I wallowed in the majesty of high church, statues of beauty, frescoes and gold that bury my lustreless drab Presbyterianism. The glory of God demands our best in every sense. I want more of it.

Another atom splitting moment was in the Capella degli Scrovegni. Here I saw the frescoes of Giotto. The depiction of heaven, hell and damnation dominate one wall, seen by the worshippers as they left the chapel. Peasants in past centuries unable to read saw the message clearly.

Saturday was given to Vicenza, the city of Palladio, the Golden City. Here was another explosion in the mind – the Olympic Theatre, Palladio's last masterpiece.

Work began on this in February 1580, but Palladio died a few months later. It is a semi-elliptical theatre with the stage in the shape of a triumphal arch, and has the tripartite form of the grand façades of Palladian palaces. The structure is plastered brick and the statues were made of plaster. Seven streets to represent the city of Thebes enter the stage. This stage though limited for performance is indeed a work of art.

Sunday was spent in the Venice Laguna. Burano island with its multicoloured houses and streets decked with the local lace looks across to St Mark's square, with the real time image of a Canaletto.

In Torcello island we saw the Cattedrale built in 639 and had lunch in Locanda Cipriani, a favourite haunt of Ernest Hemingway. Lunch finished we took the boat to Marco Polo Airport. Fully satisfied but sad to leave we boarded the British Airways plane. The food on board of hard bread roll, tasteless ham and stale cheese signalled we had indeed left Italy.

The celebration in London began on Thursday 20th June. London committee members entertained Professor Thiene, Dr C. Basso and colleagues to a dinner in the Athenaeum, a fitting welcome for the Italian committee. On Friday 21st June, eighty delegates were welcomed to a symposium in Lettsom House, Chandos Street, London on behalf of the Royal College of Physicians, the Harveian Society of London and the Medical Society of London. I took the chair in the morning and Dr Michael O'Brien, immediate Past President, officiated in the afternoon. The symposium 'Harvey and his Legacy', covered the history of medicine at the time of Harvey, the prevention of heart disease and the development of the physiology of the circulation. Professor Ian McDonald, Harveian Librarian of the Royal College of Physicians, gave an introduction to the Harvey Exhibition to be displayed in the College that evening.

Following the symposium there was a formal dinner at the Royal College of Physicians attended by 140 delegates, of which forty were from Padua. Among the guests were the Master of the Worshipful Society of Apothecaries of London, the President of the Medical Society of London and the President of the Hunterian Society. As President of The Harveian Society of London, I proposed the toast to Harvey, which was taken in silence, as is the custom. Sir George Alberti proposed the health of the guests and Professor Sergio Dalla Volta of the University of Padua replied. The diners enjoyed good food, good wine and good company. It was a successful evening in every respect.

On Saturday 22nd June, delegates boarded two coaches for Hempstead and Cambridge. Our first stop was to be at Hempstead church in Essex, built of seventeenth-century brick and containing the tomb of Harvey in the Harvey chapel, and indeed a number of monuments to the Harvey family whose estates were in this county. The church in a pleasant rural setting, contrasts with the hustle and bustle of the twenty-first century. Here sits a modest tomb for a man who changed the world of medicine. This is not a seat of academia or a princely shrine, but in this place is a peace which prompts silent prayer and meditation.

We next boarded the coaches to proceed to Cambridge. Our Italian visitors, coming from their ancient University and the environs of celebrated Palladian towns, savoured the beauty of the winding leafy lanes of the Essex countryside leading to the architectural riches of the Cambridge colleges with their tranquil manicured lawns and cloistered courts. We inhaled the atmosphere of Caius court and passed through the college's famous gates of Humility, Virtue and Honour. Delegates enjoyed a conducted tour of Gonville and Caius, including a visit to the library where a large collection of ancient manuscripts was on view.

Lunch was taken at Trinity presided over by the Deputy Master who gave a speech of welcome followed by a reply from Dr John Bennett. Following lunch delegates enjoyed a conducted tour of Trinity.

There was time to savour the atmosphere of this university town, walk by the river, heavy with punts and long poled youths, and stroll among stalls in craft market squares. The warm sun-soaked air was heavy with the ghosts of centuries of students and scholars. Too soon we had to board the coaches to return to London.

Early on Sunday 23rd June, delegates again packed the coaches at the Royal College of Physicians and the beauty of Regent's Park was left behind as we drove along traffic laden, graffiti embellished streets towards the motorway to Folkestone. Inside the coaches was an atmosphere of pleasant anticipation for the ceremony that was to mark the finale of our celebrations. Before that, lunch was to be taken at the Harvey Grammar School, founded in 1674 by Sir Eliab Harvey, nephew of William Harvey. The initial school roll of twenty students and one master was now a community of nine hundred students and fifty teachers. The arrangements for lunch were made by Mr John Smith, President of the Harvey Association of Folkestone and a past pupil of the school. The lunch was attended by the deputy headmaster. The room was graced by a painting of Harvey and the tables held crossed flags of Italy and the United Kingdom. A speech of welcome was made by Mr John Smith, part of which was in Italian. A vote of thanks was given by me on behalf of the Harveian Society of London, the Medical Society of London and the Royal College of Physicians.

Following lunch the coaches left for the Burlington Hotel close to the shore at Folkestone. Delegates were met by the Mayor, the Charter Trustees of Folkestone, city dignitaries including the Town Clerk and the chaplain. Academic gowns were worn for the procession along the promenade to the Harvey statue where wreaths were to be laid. Our Italian colleagues, resplendent in colourful robes, many medieval in

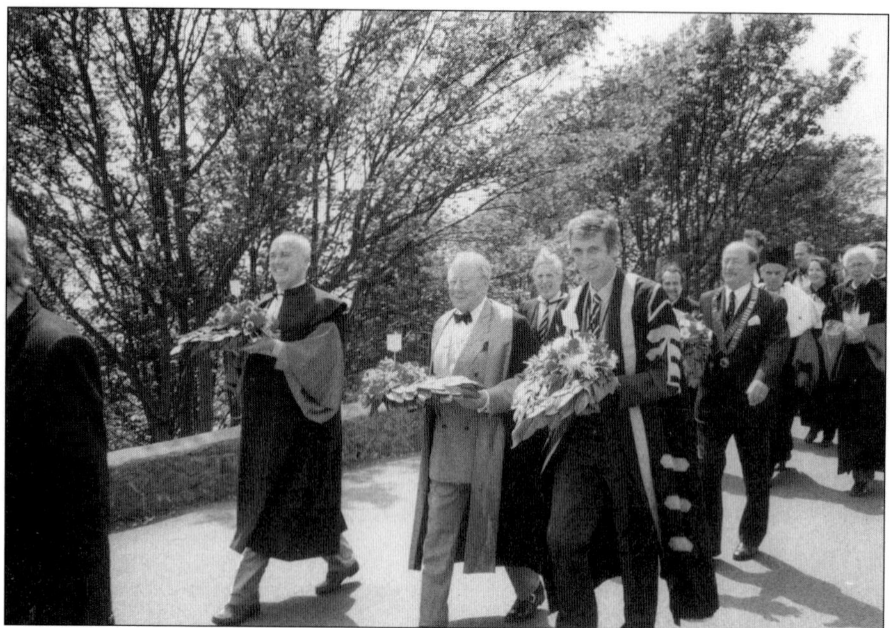

Left to right Professor Thiene, the author, and Sir George Alberti, President Royal College of Physicians, in the parade to lay wreaths at Harvey's Memorial in Folkestone

design, and bright hats of varying shapes, added grandeur to the occasion. A band in the stand on the promenade played the Harvey March as we passed. (I was unaware that such a March existed and am still unaware of its origin.)

Wreaths were laid by the Mayor, the President of the Harvey Association of Folkestone, Professor Thiene for Padua University, the President of the Royal College of Physicians, the President of the Harveian Society of London and Colonel Kinsella-Bevan for the Medical Society of London. Prayers were said by the chaplain. The Mayor and Charter Trustees entertained the delegates to a traditional English tea of scones, cream and jam at the Burlington Hotel. A welcoming speech was made by the Mayor, who also gave part of his address in Italian. I gave a vote of thanks to the Mayor and Charter Trustees.

The Italian delegates boarded the coach for Gatwick airport tired but well satisfied with the dignity of the celebrations and the warmth of the welcome they had experienced. We bade them *buon viaggio* with handshakes and hugs before returning to London content that all had gone well.

Chapter 22

Physicians, Prose and Poetry

The president of the Harveian Society of London is required to give a Presidential address for the last meeting of the year in which he presides. I had many conflicting thoughts as to the subject I should choose, but following my interest in writing decided something relating to literature would be appropriate. I was certain that I didn't wish to speak on a medical topic as such but if the two could be combined in some way I would be delighted. After deliberating for some time I choose my subject and reproduce the address here.

Physicians, Prose and Poetry

When the pre-medical course was abandoned at St Mary's Hospital Medical School and others, when students were required to sit their A levels in the sciences for entry to medical schools, I thought it an unwise decision. I thought the exclusion of the classics and art subjects as an entry into medical schools was a retrograde step. Sir David Smithers in 1989 wrote, 'an interest in and some appreciation of the arts is an advantage and perhaps a necessity in the successful understanding in science'. Perhaps this is an overstrong view but it was widely held prior to and in the eighteenth century. Dr Thomas Withers wrote, 'The character of a physician ought to be that of a gentleman which cannot be maintained with dignity but by a man of letters'.

No one would argue that the character of a physician ought to be that of a gentleman and today that of a gentlewoman but in 1951 Bernice Hamilton wrote 'the real point at issue was whether the education of a gentleman was necessary to a physician or merely ornamental'.

Harry Stevens, a physician of the family of Steven's Ink, wrote of Keats on passing the examination of the Court of Apothecaries, 'he surprised us all by passing – his knowledge of the classics helped a great deal'.

Smithers in his book *This Idle Trade*, wrote that more doctors had achieved fame in literature than have members of other professions.

Thomas Munro mentions 135 medical poets and prose writers. Dr Charles Dana of New York mentions 162 medical men writers of poetry. The list continues to grow.

Some of our famous medical authors continued to practise medicine. Four were physicians to kings and queens, William Denton, John Arbuthnot, Sir David Hamilton and Mark Akenside. Oliver Wendell Holmes was Professor of Anatomy at Harvard. Sir William Wilde and Oliver St John Gogarty were successful surgeons. Charles Lever and Conan Doyle were successful general practitioners.

Chekov wrote, 'Medicine is my lawful wife, and literature my mistress. When I get tired of one, I spend the night with other – neither of them loses anything from my infidelity'.

Many abandoned medicine for literature. Smollett, a medical author referring to a doctor in his book *Peregrine Pickle* wrote, 'It has been supposed that his want of success in a profession where merit cannot always insure fame or affluence was owing to his failure to render himself agreeable to the fair sex, whose favour is certainly of consequence to all candidates for eminence whether in physic or divinity'. Some were unhappy in medicine, Keats was one and Somerset Maugham another. Our medical writers were not dull. Robert Seymour Bridges became Poet Laureate. Two doctors, Latham and Morley became Professors of English Literature in University College London.

Andrew Boorde wrote to Thomas Cromwell, secretary to Cardinal Wolsey, 'Trust you no Skott, for they wyll youse flattering wordes and all ys falshode'.

Charles Lever wrote Dublin ballads and sang them in the streets.

> Wi'd charmin 'pisintry upon a fruitful sod,
> Fightin' like divils for conciliation
> An' hatin' each other – for the love of God

Has anything changed?

I still wonder what a knowledge of the arts contributes to medicine – or could it be that a knowledge of medicine contributes to the arts?

Time only permits me to enlarge on a few medical authors. Lord Wavell in his anthology of prose published in 1944 prefaced it with this aphorism, 'I have gathered a posie of other men's flowers and nothing but the thread that binds them is my own'. This is certainly true of this address.

I will start with John Keats, born 1795. John Keats is described by Louis Nesbit as one of England's greatest poets and by Smithers as a poet of the greatest brilliance. Some doubt has been expressed as to whether Keats obtained a medical degree. The facts are that in 1815 to prevent unqualified practice, all had to pass the new Court of Examiners after five years apprenticeship and a minimum of six months hospital training. Keats was apprenticed when aged 15 to Thomas Hammond. After five years he entered Guy's Hospital. At the time Guy's and St Thomas's Hospitals were combined for teaching and known as the United Hospitals. (This has a familiar ring and makes me think we go round in circles!) Sir Astley Cooper who first described the pectineal ligament lectured in anatomy and physiology at the time and he placed Keats under his own dresser. In 1816 Keats passed the examination of the Court of Apothecaries. One year later his first book of poems was published, but didn't sell well. His poems were severely criticized by the reviewers of the time. Having spent six years in medicine Keats was disillusioned and wished to spend his time with literature. He wrote 'my last operation was the opening of a man's temporal artery. I did it with the utmost nicety, but reflecting on what had passed through my mind at the time, my dexterity seemed a miracle and I never took up the lancet again'. The reviewers advised the poet when he abandoned medicine, 'to stick to your ointments, plasters and pills'. In 1818 he nursed his brother Tom who died of tuberculosis aged 19. The following year Keats wrote *La Belle Dame sans Merci*, *The Eve of St Agnes* and the *Ode to Psyche*. Keats developed an illness for which he took mercury. It has been suggested that this was syphilis, but Smithers says there is little evidence for this and it was most likely gonorrhoea. Keats had a love affair with Mrs Isabella Jones but became engaged to Fanny Brawne. Later, distressed with Fanny having a good time in London without him, he took laudanum for his misery. This reminds me of the first few lines of the *Ode to a Nightingale*,

> My heart aches, and a drowsy numbness pains
> My sense as though of hemlock I had drunk,
> Or emptied some dull opiate to the drains
> One minute past.

In 1820 Keats had his first haemoptysis. Fanny and her mother nursed him until he went to Italy with Joseph Severn, the artist, with whom he shared rooms at the foot of the Spanish Steps in Rome. Severn nursed him affectionately until his death aged 26.

Blackwoods noted his premature death as that of 'a young man who left a decent calling for the melancholy trade of Cockney poetry'. How wrong this has proved to be.

Severn returned to Rome 40 years later as British Consul and lived to be 86. He is buried beside Keats in Rome.

Oliver Goldsmith born 1730: I should know him well, as I passed his statue every day where it stands outside Trinity College, Dublin.

His statue doesn't show the disfigurement of his face, pitted by smallpox when he was eight years old. It cannot show his kindness and sympathy, his constant debt yet giving what little he had to poor families. He was described as foolish, impulsive and boastful. A lover of fine and colourful clothes but constantly in debt to his tailor. Gogarty describes him as 'the gentle Irish Virgil'. Boswell wrote, 'a pedantic fellow with some genius'. He was descended from a Roman Catholic priest who became a Protestant minister. His father was the Reverend Charles Goldsmith. His father's brother-in-law, the Rev. Thomas Contarine was the grandson of a Venetian aristocrat who ran away from Italy with a nun whom he married. This uncle supported Oliver as best he could with an allowance. Oliver entered Trinity College, Dublin in 1744 but three years later sold his books and ran away to Cork because of chastisement by his tutor. He returned and obtained his BA in 1749. As a student he wrote ballads which he sold profitably. Having obtained his BA his uncle gave him £50 and he set off for London to study law at the Temple. He never arrived, having only got as far as Dublin, where he lost all his money gambling. Desperate, his uncle sent him to study medicine in Edinburgh. Here he again got into debt but was rescued by fellow Irish students. He failed to qualify and decided to go to Leiden. On the way he was arrested and imprisoned in Newcastle, suspected of recruiting for the French. On reaching Leiden his luck at gambling improved and he won some money and moved to Padua for six months. While there his uncle died and his allowance ceased. He returned in 1756 to run a medical practice in Bankside, south of London Bridge. He said he had a degree from Padua and his friends thought he had one from Dublin. In 1769 Oxford gave him an MB ad eundem as they thought he was already a medical graduate of Dublin.

Soon he began to move in literary circles and ceased to practise when he joined the staff of *The Monthly Review* on a salary of £100 a year plus board and lodging. He next wrote for *The Critical Review*. At the age of 30 he was an acknowledged writer and among his friends counted Garrick, Reynolds and Samuel Johnson. Johnson tells the story of 'The Bottle of Madeira'.

> I received one morning a message from poor Goldsmith that he was in great distress and as it was not in his power to come to me, begging that I should come to him as soon as possible. I sent him a guinea and promised to come to him directly. I accordingly went as soon as I was 'drest' and found that his landlady had arrested him for his rent, at which he was in violent passion. I perceived that he had already changed my guinea and had a bottle of Madeira and a glass before him. I put the cork in the bottle, desired he should be calm and began to talk to him of the means by which he might be extricated. He then told me he had a novel ready for the press which he produced to me. I looked into it and saw its merits; told the landlady I should soon return and having gone to a bookseller sold it for £60. I brought Goldsmith the money and he discharged his rent, not without rating his landlady in a high tone for having used him so ill.

So it was that Johnson was the first person to read and appreciate *The Vicar of Wakefield*.

Goldsmith continued to produce wide ranging works including the play *She Stoops to Conquer* dedicated to Johnson.

Goldsmith was acknowledged as a genius, a poet, playwright and an essayist. At his death he was still in debt. A monument was erected to him in Westminster Abbey and Johnson wrote a Latin inscription saying, '*Nullum quod tetigit non ornavit*'. (There is almost no kind of writing that he did not touch: none that he touched he did not adorn.)

Three other Irish medical writers are worthy of attention, Charles Lever, Sir William Wilde and Oliver St John Gogarty.

Lever, born in 1806, a graceful dancer, swordsman, horseman and story-teller practised medicine in Ireland and then in Brussels. In Canada he was admitted to the Fellowship of a Red Indian tribe. He had a good medical reputation among the aristocrats and diplomats and wrote extensively, 30 books in 35 years. His books were said to record many exciting incidents, historical scenes and a great deal of Irish humour. One of Lever's friends was Thackeray who dedicated his Irish Sketch Book to him. Lever was appointed Consul in Trieste by Lord Derby who said, 'Here is £600 a year for doing nothing and you Lever, are the very man to do it.' Lever was a close friend of Sir William Wilde, born 1815, Oscar's father.

Wilde was a better doctor than Lever and was apprenticed to Abraham Colles and taught by Robert Graves and William Stokes of Stokes Adams and Cheyne Stokes fame. While I was a student in the Meath Hospital in Dublin I was on the team of Mr Stokes, an elderly surgeon descendent of William Stokes, and I had the privilege of assisting him at an operation, which I remember was a partial thyroidectomy. I also remember that in the hospital he was always accompanied by his pet dog, a small wire haired terrier.

Wilde, having taken the Licence of the Royal College of Surgeons in Ireland, studied in London at Moorfields Hospital and specializing in ophthalmology set up St Mark's Hospital in Dublin on the style of Moorfields. He was the principal surgeon. He set up practice in Dublin in 1838 and was elected to the Royal Irish Academy one year later, having earned a reputation as a speaker to learned societies. Wilde travelled extensively and wrote a series of articles for the Dublin University magazine and an account of his travels. He published a book on the literary life and scientific institutions of Austria and later toured Europe and wrote on museum antiquities and archeological research.

Wilde had a major problem – women. Smithers refers to this as Wilde's joy. The target of his sexual appetite was therefore unlike that of his son Oscar. William Wilde had three illegitimate children before marriage, not all to the same woman, a son and two daughters. The fate of the daughters was to be tragic. When aged 21 and 23 while dancing at a ball the crinoline dress of one brushed the fire and caught alight. The second daughter rushing to her aid suffered the same mishap and both died.

Wilde married Jane Francesca Elgee who wrote poetry under the pseudonym of Speranza and strongly nationalistic essays under the pseudonym of John Fenshaw Ellis. They had two sons, Willie and Oscar and a daughter Isola.

Wilde's hospital thrived and he became a leading medical figure in Europe before the age of 40. When he was at the height of his fame he saw a patient, Mary Travers aged 19, the neurotic daughter of the Professor of Medical Jurisprudence in Trinity College. She became his mistress. When he tried to discard her some time later, she created a public scandal, forcing him to take action against her in the courts. She was unimpressive in court, changing her evidence and making accusations of his using chloroform and even trying to choke her. The judge disbelieved her but the jury found in her favour but only awarded one farthing in damages. Wilde was devastated and additionally having lost his legitimate daughter Isola he became dispirited and his last years were unhappy. The court case marked a turning point in his career, as did the court case for his son Oscar some years later.

Wilde's illegitimate son, Henry Wilson qualified as a doctor and took over St Mark's Hospital from his father who retired to the country. Sir William died in 1876 aged 61. As he lay dying he was visited each day by a woman dressed in black and veiled who sat beside his bed without speaking. She has never been identified but I long to think that this may have been Mary Travers . . . but come to be forgiven or to gloat, we will never know. Wilde's funeral was attended by the President and Council of the Royal Irish Academy.

Among the most colourful of our medical authors in the twentieth century was Oliver St John Gogarty born in 1878.

A portrait was painted by Augustus John and others were painted by Sir William Orpen and Gerard Brockenhurst. His was a personality larger than life, a story teller, a *bon viveur* and a wit. Yeats wrote of him, 'I think him one of the great lyric poets of our age', but Yeats is accused of overvaluing Gogarty's poetry.

It is said that Gogarty's major work lies in his *Collected Poems* published as late as 1951. Yeats included 17 of Gogarty's poems in the *Oxford Book of Modern Verse* in 1936. Smithers says, 'Gogarty never achieved the heights of his profession or the full recognition of his literary worth; people famous for their wit have difficulty in acquiring the highest level of regard from their contemporaries, whether in art, administration or scholarship.'

Gogarty, whose father and grandfather were doctors, was born in a caul, a sign of good luck in Irish folklore. He was educated by the

Jesuits in Stonyhurst and Clongowes Wood in Ireland. He studied medicine in Trinity College Dublin, qualifying in 1907 aged 29. He was a keen athelete and swimmer, the latter saving his life some years later. He was a cyclist, a horseman and later in life owned and flew his own aeroplane. He was a wild youth and a friend of James Joyce who used him as the model for Buck Mulligan in Ulysses.

Gogarty decided to specialize in ENT surgery and spent some time training in London. He wrote about this, saying, 'Here the doctors are so kind and professional, conduct is so nice that they never contradict each other. To maintain this harmony it is taboo to make a diagnosis.'

In Dublin he joined the staff of the Richmond Hospital, (incidentally where my wife did her internship); he bought a house just off St Stephen's Green, (a prestigious part of the city), and a butter coloured Rolls Royce. He said, 'I'm going to drive myself into a successful practice'.

An opera singer came to see him having lost his voice. Gogarty diagnosed hysterical aphonia. Peering down the man's throat Gogarty said, 'I see both your parents had syphilis . . .' 'They did not,' roared the singer. 'You're cured,' roared Gogarty.

The red light district of Dublin was known as 'the kips'. Gogarty wrote of Joyce,

> There is a young fellow named Joyce,
> Who possesseth a sweet tenor voice,
> He goes to the kips,
> With a psalm on his lips,
> And biddeth the harlots rejoice.

In fact Joyce did have a good tenor voice and came second to John McCormick in the Feis Coel in Dublin. Gogarty, conscious of the poor living in tenement slums in Dublin, wrote three plays about tenement life which were produced in the Abbey Theatre and were forerunners of those by Sean O'Casey.

Gogarty had an interest in politics and wished to better the lives of the poor. He became a senator in the Irish Free State after the rebellion but when this was followed by civil war, he became a marked man. He successfully hid Michael Collins in his house when the disenchanted in the IRA came to kill him. Later Gogarty himself was taken to be shot. In freezing December he dived fully clothed into the River Liffey and under a hail of bullets swam to safety. He vowed he would present swans to the river if he escaped alive. In 1925 in company with President Cosgrave and the poet Yeats he launched a pair of swans from the boathouse of Trinity College on to the river and then published a book of poems, *An Offering of Swans*. In 1936, the year his poems were published by Yeats, Gogarty produced his book, *As I was Going Down Sackville Street*, and two years later his novel *Tumbling in the Hay* about his student days.

Horace Reynolds writing a foreword in *Others to Adorn*, in 1938 by Gogarty says,

> Three years passed and it so happened that each year I met an Irish poet who had known Gogarty, Joseph Campbell, James Stevens and Padraic Colum, and from each I gleaned something of the famous Dublin doctor. To ask of him was to evoke a legend, 'He does not belong to our spindling self-nauseated age, he is a buck of the robust, devil may care eighteenth century, born out of time to our delight'. He describes meeting Gogarty – 'I turned to see him coming toward me, eyes laughing, step quick, all smile and gaiety and good spirits, a very young middle aged man – Oliver St John Gogarty in the flesh. President Cosgrave came in, a quiet sober man who unlike most Irishmen did not want centre stage. He talked little, I fear I listened less.
>
> What were presidents to me – I sat in the presence of Gogarty.

In his poetry Gogarty broods on beauty and often female beauty. Here is an extract from one of his poems,

To the Maids not to walk in the Wind

When the wind blows, walk not abroad,
For maids, you may not know
The mad quaint thoughts which incommode
Me when the winds do blow.

But when your clothes reveal your thighs
And surge around your knees
Until from foam you seem to rise
Like Venus from the seas.

In 1939 Gogarty tried to join the British Armed Forces at the outbreak of the second world war. He was rejected as he was 62 years old. He went on an extended lecture tour of America where later he died of a heart attack in 1957. His last words were 'I think my trouble is coming on me'. These were the words first used by Yeats regarding his love for Maud Gonne McBride.

Initially in this address I intended to look at the lives of Sir Arthur Conan Doyle born in 1893, and Somerset Maugham born in 1974, but time permits me only a cursory consideration. There are features about their lives which illustrate the kernel of my belief regarding the bond between physicians, prose and poetry.

Sir Arthur Conan Doyle, qualified in Edinburgh and influenced by one of his teachers, Dr Bell, created Sherlock Holmes, who later was to plague him. He said 'A monstrous growth has come out of what was really a comparatively small seed. As to the people who write to Holmes care of the author I wish they would leave me alone'. Conan Doyle was a catholic who rejected Catholicism, who for a time was an atheist, and next a spiritualist. He wrote seven books on spiritualism. In 1893 he said, ' I am in the middle of my last Holmes story'. He was to write others later but feared he was to be associated with what he considered a lower stratum of literary achievement. However there is little doubt that the successful writing of Conan Doyle was greatly influenced by his medical training and clinical background.

Somerset Maugham trained at St Thomas's Hospital. I think the best painting of him was by Sutherland. He and Conan Doyle considered themselves story tellers. This they were, and indeed Somerset Maugham was the best selling medical story teller ever. Frederick Raphael in a review in the *Times Literary Supplement* said, 'He was a man who put his cards on the table better to conceal the ace up his sleeve'. His first book, *Liza of Lambeth*, written when he was 23, was based on his experience as a medical student in the slums of Lambeth. It didn't sell well. His masterpiece, *Of Human Bondage*, is the story of his first thirty years of life and includes his period of medical training.

In my opening paragraphs I referred to the concept in the past centuries that to be a good doctor required a literary education. I wish to leave you tonight with a mirror-image view that a medical education is fertile ground for literary ambition. It was said that Keats was a member of the medical profession, the members of which in common with most artists understand compassion and exercise critical discernment about intensely personal concerns. Sampson Handley in an introductory address at the Middlesex Hospital in 1913 said, 'The personal services which a medical student gives to the more unfortunate of his fellow citizens, the intimate contact he makes with their miseries and heroisms, virtues and vices must tend to broaden his outlook on life.'

A.M. Cooke, physician, Emeritus Fellow of Merton College, Oxford wrote in 1974, 'The medical student learns about man, not only his anatomy, physiology, psychology and pathology but his environment, his work and play, his hopes and fears, and perhaps more importantly about the seamy side of man's nature'.

Louis Nesbit writing on Physicians of the Past and Present, in 1935 said, 'The physician's daily routine places him in most intimate touch with human nature, He knows better than other men the innermost soul of his fellow man. He of all men should have a message to deliver to the world'.

I am anxious that today, with the emphasis on science, clinical studies and clinical analysis may diminish, and we may not touch the innermost soul of our fellow man. Reading outside our scientific texts may also diminish. As long ago as 1893, William Banks in an address to the Medical Society of London said, 'So completely did my medical reading crush out of me all desire for general literature that it was long after I graduated ere the desire for it returned'.

Perhaps the last words reflecting my thoughts should rest in, 'The Summing up', by Somerset Maugham referring to his medical training at StThomas's Hospital. 'For here I was in contact with what I most wanted, life in the raw. In those years I must have witnessed pretty well every emotion of which man is capable. I do not know a better training for a writer than to spend some years in the medical profession.

Ladies and Gentlemen,

We here tonight have spent many years in the medical profession and in each of us lies a profound and eventful story.

Chapter 23

The Freshers Lecture

When I was the director of Clinical Studies at St Mary's Hospital Medical School, and responsible for the students and their curriculum, I gave an introductory lecture during Freshers Week. This began as a description of the curriculum, but soon I wanted to say more. Gradually I expanded this lecture into a talk on what it meant to be a medical student, what would be expected of them and especially what it meant to be a doctor, their chosen future and their responsibilities for their patients. I wanted to tell them the highest ideals to which they should strive, and that these ideals are sacred to the noble profession of medicine. This became known as 'The Freshers Lecture' and was sometimes introduced as the 'Oscar Craig' lecture.

When my time as Director of Clinical Studies ended I was requested to continue to give this talk and indeed to my surprise, although retired for eleven years I am still asked to do it. It is given now in Imperial College School of Medicine because of the merging of medical schools and each class has circa 300 students yearly. It was this lecture that figured in the series *Doctors to Be* produced by the BBC.

When I look at these young, expectant and purposeful boys and girls, my spirits are raised and I yearn for them. I want their medical lives to be fulfilled and I want them to stand for all that is best in the medical profession. If ever I drop dead, I want to do so finishing this lecture. What a time to go, at the height of doing something I believe in so strongly and when my hopes are full of the enthusiasm I see and feel in the room.

This lecture is not written, but given 'off the cuff'. It is difficult to reproduce the effect of the lecture or the enthusiasm of the Freshers merely by the written word, my skill as a writer is insufficient to do so. What you read is emphasized by repetition, gestures, smiles, frowns and indeed by shameless acting.

The Freshers Lecture

1. This is the most important day in your life. Nothing will ever be the same again. You haven't just signed on for a job – you have taken on

a new way of life, a new way of thinking, a new way of feeling, a new way of acting – you will never be the same again after you leave this room – you have taken on medicine – you have begun your path to being doctors.

There may be 300 of you in this room, but I speak to each of you individually – to you, and you and you. Look into my eyes as I look into yours. You will not have this lecture again, and you will not hear what I have to say from anyone else during your medical course.

2. Imperial College School of Medicine is a young school, composed of St Mary's, Charing Cross and Westminster schools. Each of these medical schools had a tradition of academic excellence, and excellent extra curricular activities in sports, music and drama. Each had a long and respected reputation. You have an awesome responsibility to carry these traditions to Imperial, so that Imperial College School of Medicine will have meaning and status and you can carry the badge of Imperial with pride. It is up to you and may you – walk tall.

3. The medical course has changed over the years and now at Imperial you will be introduced to patients earlier than in the past. You will meet patients in hospitals and general practice in what previously were the pre-clinical years. This is good, but I want to warn you to build your medicine on firm foundations, on rock and not sand. Do not neglect the basic sciences – anatomy, physiology and biochemistry. They are not boring and they are the basic bricks of your house. If only I had paid more attention to embryology, I would have understood congenital heart disease better in my clinical years.

In this new course you have an added year to do a BSc. Make good use of it – you will learn the value of research. Soon enough you will study surgery, general medicine, obstetrics and gynaecology and all the other specialties, rheumatology, dermatology and every other 'ology'.

You will visit many hospitals as well as the major teaching hospitals – you will visit District General hospitals in and around London – you will visit Accident and Emergency departments, and you will have an Elective Period when you can study what you wish in medicine and where you wish for some months. This may be abroad, in Africa, India, the United States of America, Europe or elsewhere or even here at home. You have to fund this part yourself, but there are scholarships and grants you may compete for. Make good use of this Elective Period – it is not a holiday.

4. Now I wish to talk to you about what I call the Graph of Enthusiasm.

At the moment you are all feeling wonderful. You have begun medicine.

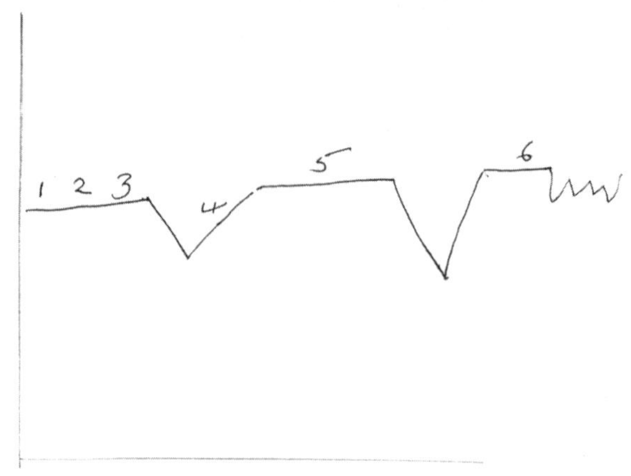

Graph of Enthusiasm

You've managed to get here. You've left home, you are in London, you can make your own decisions. The boys are meeting new girls. The girls are meeting new boys.

It's all very exciting. You are high on the graph.

This may last for some time, but after the second year you have got used to all that – even the boy/girl associations may change.

'John, how are you getting on with Jane?'

'Funny you should ask that. I'm getting worried. She's got very serious. I think she expects me to marry her. I feel trapped.'

The girls' conversation,

'Joan, how are things with Bill?'

'He's got boring. He's only after one thing, and he'll make a good surgeon, he's got hands everywhere. I'm getting tired of him.'

Also at this stage you wish to be more involved in the major subjects and more involved with patients. You are used to London, it's not so exciting. Being a medical student is not so wonderful as it was. You take a dive in your enthusiasm and a dip appears on the graph.

Later the real clinical time appears and with it your badge of office, the stethoscope.

This is important to you – you may wear it round your neck like the best necklace you ever had – the boys have it protruding from a jacket pocket, suitably visible at all times, even walking in the street. While shopping the girls may drop it from a handbag,

'Oh! You're a doctor. You're very young.'

The girls smile back but don't deny it.

At this stage in your course the graph goes up. You are again loving medicine.

Within the next year or so, it dawns on you that there is so much to learn that it's impossible. You have to spend all your time studying. The examinations are a lottery. If you can't answer the consultants they get sarcastic. You are very tired.

You can't cope with all this and the patients can be difficult. You think, why did I study medicine? What am I doing? I feel desperate. I'm in the wrong profession.

Let me tell you – you will cry. Even the boys may cry. You will be filled with doubt. You will think, I'm the only one to feel like this.

Let me tell you – we have all been there.

When this happens to you, and it may happen at different times, some early, some late, do not doubt yourself. You are not in the wrong profession. Never doubt yourself – this phase will pass. This phase will pass.

5. I made a great mistake during my medical course. I worked too hard. I didn't get the balance right. You are only a medical student once in your life.

You are only at university once in your life. Get the balance right between work and play. Too much play and you will fail your exams – too much work and you may be boring and perhaps not so good a doctor. Get the balance right. This is not easy. You should take part in the life of the school and university. Play some sports, there are many choices. Think of music, there are choirs and orchestras.

Think of dramatics. If you can't be out front, think of back stage.

Be involved and you will be a happier student. A happier student will study better.

A happier individual is a better doctor.

6. What makes you a good doctor is largely motivation. The motives that made you want to be a doctor in your youth are the correct motives. Never forget them and never be ashamed of your youthful

motives. If you wished to do medicine to help human beings or to improve the quality of life for others, then what is wrong with that? Stick to your early motives. You will need these motives when times are hard, and hard times will come.

Your greatest strength today is – your youth. You are not cluttered with negative thoughts – it all lies before you – never doubt yourself and never let anyone rubbish your youth.

You are a chosen people to be here at all – feel confident about what you wish to do – and go for it.

7. When you qualify you will face problems. Remember above all that medicine is about people; people like your father, mother, brother, sister, cousin.

You may cry again from tiredness, frustration, anxiety, temper, disappointment, pity and you may suffer from medical litigation. Through all this remember that people need you in their hour of pain, anxiety and stress.

There is nothing in this world more important than one human being – no matter how lowly. For every human being you must display competence and compassion.

Remember the value of holding a hand. There may be times when all you can do is hold a patient's hand. Do not neglect to do so. Remember what I say today. The future of medicine is in your hands.

8. I can sum up with the words of Christina Rossetti:

> Will the road wind uphill all the way?
> Yes, to the very end.
> Will the day's journey take the whole long day?
> From morn till night, my friend.

I cannot leave it on that note alone, so I wrote a piece I call 'After Rossetti:

> Will there be no joy, no hope, no success?
> To overfill your cup my friend,
> To overfill your cup.

So – Rise up with wings as eagles, run and not weary,
And – May your God go with you.

Index of names

Entries in italics indicate an illustration